The Anti-Inflammatory Smoothie Cookbook

Easy, Mouthwatering and Nutritious Smoothie Recipes to Reduce Inflammation, Boost Your Immune System, and Enhance Wellness. Includes a 30-Day Meal Plan

Amanda K. Sanders

Table of Contents

Introduction to the Anti-Inflammatory Smoothie Diet

Understanding Inflammation

Inflammation is a natural response of the body's immune system to injury, infection, or harmful stimuli. The biological process is complex, requiring the activation of immune cells, the release of signaling molecules, and increased blood flow to the affected area. This process is crucial for promoting healing and safeguarding the body from additional damage. However, if inflammation persists over time, it can lead to various health problems such as heart disease, diabetes, arthritis, and certain cancers.

Acute inflammation is a temporary condition that usually goes away once the body has successfully addressed the threat at hand. The condition is marked by redness, swelling, heat, and pain at the location of injury or infection. However, chronic inflammation is a long-lasting, low-grade inflammation that continues for an extended period, often without any noticeable symptoms. Various factors, including an unhealthy diet, high stress levels, lack of physical activity, and exposure to environmental toxins, can contribute to its development.

Benefits of an Anti-Inflammatory Diet

An anti-inflammatory diet emphasizes eating foods that reduce inflammation and promote general health. This diet focuses on whole, nutrient-dense foods packed with antioxidants, vitamins, minerals, and healthy fats. By adding anti-inflammatory foods to your daily routine, you can enjoy a wide range of health benefits, including:

1. **Reduced Risk of Chronic Diseases**: Eating an anti-inflammatory diet will help reduce your chance of developing chronic diseases like heart disease, diabetes, and certain cancers. This is accomplished by reducing inflammation, enhancing blood sugar regulation, and promoting cardiovascular health.

2. **Improved Digestive Health:** Foods with anti-inflammatory properties, particularly those rich in fiber, contribute to a balanced gut microbiome and enhance digestion. This can provide relief for symptoms of digestive disorders like irritable bowel syndrome (IBS) and inflammatory bowel disease (IBD).

3. **Optimal Immune Function:** A diet rich in antioxidants and essential nutrients promotes a robust immune system, enabling your body to combat infections and illnesses better.

4. **Improved Weight Management:** Following an anti-inflammatory diet can support better regulation of body weight through the inclusion of nutrient-rich, low-calorie foods. This can help reduce the risk of obesity, which is a major contributor to chronic inflammation and associated diseases.

5. **Relief from Joint Pain and Inflammation:** Consuming anti-inflammatory foods can reduce joint pain and swelling and relieve symptoms of arthritis and other inflammatory conditions.

<u>Why You Need Anti-Inflammatory Juices and Smoothies</u>

Anti-inflammatory juices and smoothies are an easy and delightful way to add inflammation-fighting foods into your diet. They provide numerous benefits, making them valuable to your everyday routine. Below are some of the benefits of taking anti-inflammatory smoothies and juices:

1. **Rich in Nutrients:** Juices and smoothies are high in vitamins, minerals, antioxidants, and phytonutrients, all of which help in reducing inflammation. By combining fruits, vegetables, nuts, seeds, and herbs, a potent anti-inflammatory beverage can be crafted to nourish your body.

2. **Efficient Digestion and Absorption:** Blending fruits and vegetables effectively breaks down their cell walls, allowing your body to absorb their valuable nutrients efficiently. This is particularly helpful for people who experience digestive problems, as it lessens the strain on the digestive system and enables faster absorption of nutrients.

3. **Hydration:** Numerous ingredients known for their anti-inflammatory properties, including cucumbers, berries, and citrus fruits, have high water content. Beverages like freshly made juices and smoothies are great for staying hydrated, which is crucial for overall health and supporting your body's natural detoxification processes.

4. **Convenience:** Juices and smoothies are convenient for busy people due to their quick and easy preparation. They're ideal for a quick breakfast, a post-workout snack, or a refreshing midday pick-up.

5. **Versatility:** The options for making anti-inflammatory juices and smoothies are limitless. You can experiment with different combinations of fruits, vegetables, herbs, and spices to suit your taste and nutritional requirements.

6. **Embrace a Healthy Lifestyle:** Including anti-inflammatory juices and smoothies in your diet can lead to healthier eating habits. They can act as a springboard for discovering more anti-inflammatory foods and recipes, allowing you to develop a long-term approach to health and wellness.

In conclusion, understanding inflammation and its effects on health is critical for making sound dietary choices. By embracing an anti-inflammatory diet and integrating nutrient-rich juices and smoothies into your daily routine, you can strengthen your body's innate healing abilities, lower your risk of chronic diseases, and enhance your overall health.

Chapter 1: Helpful Tips for Successful Anti-Inflammatory Juicing

Choosing the Right Ingredients

Selecting the right ingredients is crucial for crafting potent anti-inflammatory juices and smoothies. Here are some helpful tips for choosing the highest quality produce to enhance your health:

1. **Choose Fresh, Whole Foods:** Give preference to fresh, whole fruits and vegetables instead of processed or pre-packaged choices. Fresh produce is known for its high nutrient content and better anti-inflammatory benefits. Whenever possible, choose organic produce to reduce exposure to pesticides and chemicals that may worsen inflammation.

2. **Focus on Antioxidant-Rich Ingredients:** Incorporating ingredients that are rich in antioxidants can help combat oxidative stress and reduce inflammation. These include a variety of berries (blueberries, strawberries, raspberries), dark leafy greens (kale, spinach), and brightly colored vegetables (bell peppers, carrots).

3. **Add Healthy Fats:** Incorporating healthy fats into your diet is vital for reducing inflammation. Avocados, nuts, seeds, and coconut oil are all great sources of these healthy fats. Adding a modest quantity of these fats into your juices and smoothies can improve the absorption of nutrients and give them a delightful, smooth consistency.

4. **Spice It Up:** Incorporate anti-inflammatory spices and herbs like turmeric, ginger, cinnamon, and mint into your recipes. These impressive additions not only enhance flavor but also have potent anti-inflammatory benefits.

5. **Be Mindful of the Sugars:** Although fruits are essential to anti-inflammatory juicing, it is critical to balance their natural sugars. Combine sweet fruits with low-sugar veggies such as cucumbers, celery, and leafy greens to keep blood sugar levels constant and avoid unnecessary spikes.

6. **Include Fiber-Rich Ingredients:** Fiber promotes digestive health and maintains inflammation levels. Adding ingredients such as chia seeds, flaxseeds, and oats to your smoothies can provide a good source of fiber and contribute to a healthier gut and overall well-being.

Balancing Flavors and Nutrients

Crafting a wholesome anti-inflammatory juice or smoothie that is both nourishing and delightful demands careful consideration of flavors and nutrients. Here are some tips to help you in achieving the perfect balance:

1. **Mix Sweet and Savory:** Achieve a perfect balance of flavors by combining sweet fruits with savory vegetables. For instance, you can combine apples or berries with spinach or kale to achieve a harmonious blend of sweetness and earthy undertones.

2. **Layer Flavors:** Enhance the complexity of your smoothies by layering different flavors to create a more dynamic taste experience. To brighten the flavor, add a hint of citrus (lemon, lime, or orange), or use a few fresh herbs like basil or cilantro for a refreshing twist.

3. **Mind the Texture:** The texture of your smoothie is just as crucial as the flavor. Use a blend of thick and liquid ingredients to attain the desired consistency. Consider incorporating ingredients such as avocado, banana, or Greek yogurt to achieve a smoother consistency. For a lighter and more refreshing beverage, consider using water, coconut water, or unsweetened almond milk.

4. **Ensure Macronutrient Balance:** Strive for a well-rounded combination of carbohydrates, proteins, and fats in your smoothies. Fruits and vegetables are a great source of carbohydrates that can give you a quick boost of energy. Greek yogurt, protein powder, nuts, avocados, and seeds are all excellent sources of protein and healthy fats that can help keep you feeling full and satisfied.

5. **Experiment with Superfoods:** Superfoods such as spirulina, chlorella, acai, and maca powder can enhance the nutritional value of your smoothies. These ingredients contain various beneficial compounds that promote good health and help decrease inflammation.

Storage and Preparation Tips

Your anti-inflammatory juices and smoothies' freshness and nutritional quality rely heavily on proper preparation and storage. Follow these tips to ensure you get the most out of your ingredients:

1. **Prep in Advance:** Be efficient by preparing your ingredients ahead of time. Ensure the fruits and vegetables are properly prepared by washing, peeling, and chopping them. Afterward, store them in airtight containers in the refrigerator. Another option is to prepare smoothie packs by dividing the ingredients into individual bags and freezing them. This makes blending quick and effortless.

2. **Store Smart:** For optimal nutritional value, it's best to enjoy your juices and smoothies shortly after making them. To ensure the best storage conditions, use airtight glass containers and refrigerate the items for no more than 24-48 hours. Using lemon or lime juice can help maintain freshness.

3. **Use Frozen Ingredients:** Frozen fruits and vegetables are convenient and nutrient-rich. Freezing protects their vitamins and minerals; frozen ingredients make your smoothie thicker and colder. Make sure to use unsweetened and unprocessed frozen options.

4. **Blend Properly:** Investing in a high-quality blender is crucial to achieve smooth and consistent results. Begin by blending leafy greens and liquids thoroughly before adding fruits, vegetables, and other ingredients. This method guarantees a smoother texture and uniform mixing.

5. **Add Ingredients in the Right Order:** When adding ingredients, follow the correct order: Begin by pouring in the liquids, then proceed with the softer ingredients, such as leafy greens and bananas. Finally, add the harder ingredients, like frozen fruits and nuts. This order ensures optimal blender performance and minimizes the risk of clogging.

6. **Clean Your Equipment:** After each usage, clean your blender immediately to prevent residue from hardening and to preserve hygiene. Ensure thorough cleaning by rinsing with warm water and a small amount of dish soap. Additionally, create a solution of water and soap to effectively clean those difficult-to-access areas. Make sure to rinse thoroughly and dry right away.

You can craft delectable, nutritious anti-inflammatory juices and smoothies by carefully choosing the ingredients, ensuring a harmonious blend of flavors and nutrients, and adhering to recommended storage and preparation techniques. Adopt these practices to maximize the effectiveness of your anti-inflammatory juicing journey and savor the multitude of benefits it provides.

.

Chapter 2: 30-Day Meal Plan

Meal Plan for Days 1-30

Day	Breakfast	Lunch	Dinner
1	Berry Antioxidant Delight	Classic Green Revitalizer	Orange Turmeric Tonic
2	Blueberry Bliss	Kale and Kiwi Cleanser	Lemon Ginger Zinger
3	Raspberry Radiance	Spinach Berry Booster	Grapefruit Glow Getter
4	Blackberry Basil Boost	Cucumber Mint Magic	Lime Basil Blast
5	Strawberry Serenity	Avocado Green Dream	Citrus Carrot Crush
6	Cranberry Cool Down	Green Tea Infusion	Pineapple Citrus Sensation
7	Mixed Berry Marvel	Pineapple Spinach Pleaser	Mandarin Mango Madness
8	Pomegranate Power	Tropical Green Refresher	Lemon Lime Loveliness
9	Acai Energy Elixir	Matcha Green Energy	Citrus Berry Bliss
10	Goji Berry Glow	Broccoli Blueberry Blend	Blood Orange Beauty
11	Elderberry Immunity	Green Grapes Galore	Tangerine Tropical Twist
12	Cherry Chamomile Chill	Pear Spinach Paradise	Pomelo Passion
13	Berry Beet Blast	Celery Cilantro Cooler	Lemonade Lavender Lush
14	Citrus Berry Burst	Green Apple Ginger Zest	Citrus Cilantro Cooler
15	Mango Berry Tango	Mango Spinach Surprise	Citrus Apple Alchemy
16	Pineapple Berry Zing	Coconut Kale Craze	Citrus Kale Kicker
17	Kiwi Berry Fusion	Pea Protein Power	Orange Bell Pepper Bliss
18	Berry Banana Bliss	Watercress Cucumber Cooler	Almond Joy Delight
19	Classic Green Revitalizer	Walnut Berry Bonanza	Peanut Butter Banana Bliss
20	Kale and Kiwi Cleanser	Cashew Cinnamon Swirl	Hazelnut Chocolate Indulgence
21	Spinach Berry Booster	Pistachio Mango Madness	Macadamia Nut Marvel
22	Cucumber Mint Magic	Pecan Pie Pleaser	Brazil Nut Berry Blend

23	Avocado Green Dream	Sunflower Seed Sunshine	Sesame Ginger Glow
24	Green Tea Infusion	Flaxseed Blueberry Boost	Chia Seed Cherry Chill
25	Pineapple Spinach Pleaser	Hemp Heart Happiness	Pumpkin Seed Power
26	Tropical Green Refresher	Nutty Coconut Craze	Nutty Apricot Ambrosia
27	Matcha Green Energy	Nutty Maple Mania	Turmeric Ginger Tonic
28	Broccoli Blueberry Blend	Cinnamon Apple Delight	Ginger Pear Pleaser
29	Green Grapes Galore	Cardamom Banana Boost	Clove Orange Zest
30	Pear Spinach Paradise	Cayenne Mango Madness	Black Pepper Berry Blast

Chapter 3: Berry Blast

Berry Antioxidant Delight

Prep Time: 5 minutes | **Cook Time:** 0 minutes | **Servings:** 2

Ingredients:

- 1 cup frozen mixed berries (blueberries, strawberries, raspberries)
- 1/2 cup pomegranate juice
- 1/2 cup almond milk
- 1 tablespoon honey
- 1/2 teaspoon ground cinnamon
- 1/4 teaspoon ground ginger
- 1/4 teaspoon ground turmeric
- 1 tablespoon ground flaxseed
- 1/2 cup plain Greek yogurt
- Ice cubes (optional)

Instructions:

1. In a blender, put together the frozen mixed berries, pomegranate juice, almond milk, honey, ground cinnamon, ground ginger, ground turmeric, ground flaxseed, and plain Greek yogurt.
2. Blend until smooth.
3. If desired, add ice cubes and blend again until desired consistency is reached.
4. Pour into glasses and serve immediately.

Nutritional Information (per serving):

- **Carbs:** 25g
- **Sodium:** 45mg
- **Potassium:** 150mg
- **Protein:** 5g

Blueberry Bliss

Prep Time: 5 minutes | **Cook Time:** 0 minutes | **Servings:** 2

Ingredients:

- 1 cup frozen blueberries
- 1 ripe banana, peeled and sliced
- 1/2 cup unsweetened almond milk
- 1/2 cup plain Greek yogurt
- 1 tablespoon honey
- 1 tablespoon chia seeds
- 1/2 teaspoon vanilla extract
- 1/4 teaspoon ground cinnamon
- Ice cubes (optional)

Instructions:

1. In a blender, put together the frozen blueberries, sliced ripe banana, unsweetened almond milk, plain Greek yogurt, honey, chia seeds, vanilla extract, and ground cinnamon.
2. Blend until smooth.
3. If desired, add ice cubes and blend again until desired consistency is reached.
4. Pour into glasses and serve immediately.

Nutritional Information (per serving):

- **Carbs:** 25g
- **Sodium:** 50mg
- **Potassium:** 200mg
- **Protein:** 6g

Raspberry Radiance

Prep Time: 5 minutes | **Cook Time:** 0 minutes | **Servings:** 2

Ingredients:

- 1 cup frozen raspberries
- 1/2 cup coconut water
- 1/2 cup unsweetened coconut milk
- 1/2 cup diced pineapple
- 1 tablespoon honey
- 1 tablespoon fresh lime juice
- 1 tablespoon grated ginger
- 1/2 teaspoon ground turmeric
- 1/4 teaspoon ground black pepper
- Ice cubes (optional)

Instructions:

1. In a blender, put together the frozen raspberries, coconut water, unsweetened coconut milk, diced pineapple, honey, fresh lime juice, grated ginger, ground turmeric, and ground black pepper.
2. Blend until smooth.
3. If desired, add ice cubes and blend again until desired consistency is reached.
4. Pour into glasses and serve immediately.

Nutritional Information (per serving):

- **Carbs:** 20g
- **Sodium:** 30mg
- **Potassium:** 150mg
- **Protein:** 2g

Blackberry Basil Boost

Prep Time: 5 minutes | **Cook Time:** 0 minutes | **Servings:** 2

Ingredients:

- 1 cup frozen blackberries
- 1/2 cup unsweetened almond milk
- 1/2 cup plain Greek yogurt
- 1/4 cup fresh basil leaves
- 1 tablespoon honey
- 1 tablespoon ground flaxseed
- 1/2 teaspoon grated fresh ginger
- 1/4 teaspoon ground cinnamon
- Ice cubes (optional)

Instructions:

1. In a blender, put together the frozen blackberries, unsweetened almond milk, plain Greek yogurt, fresh basil leaves, honey, ground flaxseed, grated fresh ginger, and ground cinnamon.
2. Blend until smooth.
3. If desired, add ice cubes and blend again until desired consistency is reached.
4. Pour into glasses and serve immediately.

Nutritional Information (per serving):

- **Carbs:** 15g
- **Sodium:** 40mg
- **Potassium:** 100mg
- **Protein:** 5g

Strawberry Serenity

Prep Time: 5 minutes | **Cook Time:** 0 minutes | **Servings:** 2

Ingredients:

- 1 cup frozen strawberries
- 1/2 cup unsweetened cranberry juice
- 1/2 cup coconut water
- 1/2 ripe avocado, diced
- 1 tablespoon fresh lemon juice
- 1 tablespoon honey
- 1/4 teaspoon ground turmeric
- 1/4 teaspoon ground cinnamon
- Ice cubes (optional)

Instructions:

1. In a blender, put together the frozen strawberries, unsweetened cranberry juice, coconut water, diced ripe avocado, fresh lemon juice, honey, ground turmeric, and ground cinnamon.
2. Blend until smooth.
3. If desired, add ice cubes and blend again until desired consistency is reached.
4. Pour into glasses and serve immediately.

Nutritional Information (per serving):

- **Carbs:** 20g
- **Sodium:** 35mg
- **Potassium:** 200mg
- **Protein:** 2g

Cranberry Cool Down

Prep Time: 5 minutes | **Cook Time:** 0 minutes | **Servings:** 2

Ingredients:

- 1 cup frozen cranberries
- 1/2 cup unsweetened almond milk
- 1/2 cup coconut water
- 1/2 cup diced cucumber
- 1 tablespoon fresh mint leaves
- 1 tablespoon honey
- 1/2 teaspoon grated fresh ginger
- 1/4 teaspoon ground cinnamon
- Ice cubes (optional)

Instructions:

1. In a blender, put together the frozen cranberries, unsweetened almond milk, coconut water, diced cucumber, fresh mint leaves, honey, grated fresh ginger, and ground cinnamon.
2. Blend until smooth.
3. If desired, add ice cubes and blend again until desired consistency is reached.
4. Pour into glasses and serve immediately.

Nutritional Information (per serving):

- **Carbs:** 15g
- **Sodium:** 35mg
- **Potassium:** 150mg
- **Protein:** 1g

Mixed Berry Marvel

Prep Time: 5 minutes | **Cook Time:** 0 minutes | **Servings:** 2

Ingredients:

- 1 cup frozen mixed berries (blueberries, strawberries, raspberries)
- 1/2 cup unsweetened green tea
- 1/2 cup coconut water
- 1/2 ripe banana, sliced
- 1 tablespoon fresh lemon juice
- 1 tablespoon honey
- 1 tablespoon ground flaxseed
- Ice cubes (optional)

Instructions:

1. In a blender, put together the frozen mixed berries, unsweetened green tea, coconut water, sliced ripe banana, fresh lemon juice, honey, and ground flaxseed.
2. Blend until smooth.
3. If desired, add ice cubes and blend again until desired consistency is reached.
4. Pour into glasses and serve immediately.

Nutritional Information (per serving):

- **Carbs:** 20g
- **Sodium:** 20mg
- **Potassium:** 200mg
- **Protein:** 2g

Pomegranate Power

Prep Time: 5 minutes | **Cook Time:** 0 minutes | **Servings:** 2

Ingredients:

- 1 cup pomegranate seeds
- 1/2 cup unsweetened almond milk
- 1/2 cup coconut water
- 1/2 cup diced pineapple
- 1 tablespoon fresh lime juice
- 1 tablespoon honey
- 1/2 teaspoon grated fresh ginger
- Ice cubes (optional)

Instructions:

1. In a blender, put together the pomegranate seeds, unsweetened almond milk, coconut water, diced pineapple, fresh lime juice, honey, and grated fresh ginger.
2. Blend until smooth.
3. If desired, add ice cubes and blend again until desired consistency is reached.
4. Pour into glasses and serve immediately.

Nutritional Information (per serving):

- **Carbs:** 25g
- **Sodium:** 20mg
- **Potassium:** 150mg
- **Protein:** 1g

Acai Energy Elixir

Prep Time: 5 minutes | **Cook Time:** 0 minutes | **Servings:** 2

Ingredients:

- 2 packs frozen acai puree
- 1/2 cup unsweetened coconut milk
- 1/2 cup unsweetened almond milk
- 1/2 cup frozen strawberries
- 1 ripe banana, sliced
- 1 tablespoon honey
- 1 tablespoon ground flaxseed
- Ice cubes (optional)

Instructions:

1. In a blender, put together the frozen acai puree, unsweetened coconut milk, unsweetened almond milk, frozen strawberries, sliced ripe banana, honey, and ground flaxseed.
2. Blend until smooth.
3. If desired, add ice cubes and blend again until desired consistency is reached.
4. Pour into glasses and serve immediately.

Nutritional Information (per serving):

- **Carbs:** 30g
- **Sodium:** 25mg
- **Potassium:** 200mg
- **Protein:** 2g

Goji Berry Glow

Prep Time: 5 minutes | **Cook Time:** 0 minutes | **Servings:** 2

Ingredients:

- 1/2 cup goji berries (soaked in water for 15 minutes and drained)
- 1/2 cup unsweetened almond milk
- 1/2 cup coconut water
- 1/2 cup frozen mixed berries (blueberries, strawberries, raspberries)
- 1/2 ripe avocado, diced
- 1 tablespoon honey
- 1 tablespoon fresh lemon juice
- Ice cubes (optional)

Instructions:

1. In a blender, put together the soaked and drained goji berries, unsweetened almond milk, coconut water, frozen mixed berries, diced ripe avocado, honey, and fresh lemon juice.
2. Blend until smooth.
3. If desired, add ice cubes and blend again until desired consistency is reached.
4. Pour into glasses and serve immediately.

Nutritional Information (per serving):

- **Carbs:** 20g
- **Sodium:** 30mg
- **Potassium:** 150mg
- **Protein:** 2g

Elderberry Immunity

Prep Time: 5 minutes | **Cook Time:** 0 minutes | **Servings:** 2

Ingredients:

- 1/2 cup dried elderberries (soaked in water for 1 hour and drained)
- 1/2 cup unsweetened almond milk
- 1/2 cup coconut water
- 1/2 cup frozen blackberries
- 1/2 cup diced pineapple
- 1 tablespoon honey
- 1 tablespoon fresh lemon juice
- Ice cubes (optional)

Instructions:

1. In a blender, put together the soaked and drained dried elderberries, unsweetened almond milk, coconut water, frozen blackberries, diced pineapple, honey, and fresh lemon juice.
2. Blend until smooth.
3. If desired, add ice cubes and blend again until desired consistency is reached.
4. Pour into glasses and serve immediately.

Nutritional Information (per serving):

- **Carbs:** 20g
- **Sodium:** 30mg
- **Potassium:** 200mg
- **Protein:** 2g

Cherry Chamomile Chill

Prep Time: 5 minutes | **Cook Time:** 0 minutes | **Servings:** 2

Ingredients:

- 1 cup frozen cherries
- 1/2 cup chamomile tea, cooled
- 1/2 cup unsweetened coconut milk
- 1/2 cup plain Greek yogurt
- 1 tablespoon honey
- 1/2 teaspoon vanilla extract
- Ice cubes (optional)

Instructions:

1. In a blender, put together the frozen cherries, cooled chamomile tea, unsweetened coconut milk, plain Greek yogurt, honey, and vanilla extract.
2. Blend until smooth.
3. If desired, add ice cubes and blend again until desired consistency is reached.
4. Pour into glasses and serve immediately.

Nutritional Information (per serving):

- **Carbs:** 20g
- **Sodium:** 20mg
- **Potassium:** 150mg
- **Protein:** 5g

Berry Beet Blast

Prep Time: 5 minutes | **Cook Time:** 0 minutes | **Servings:** 2

Ingredients:

- 1/2 cup cooked and diced beets
- 1 cup mixed berries (blueberries, strawberries, raspberries)
- 1/2 cup unsweetened almond milk
- 1/2 cup coconut water
- 1 tablespoon honey
- 1 tablespoon ground flaxseed
- 1/2 teaspoon grated fresh ginger
- Ice cubes (optional)

Instructions:

1. In a blender, put together the cooked and diced beets, mixed berries, unsweetened almond milk, coconut water, honey, ground flaxseed, and grated fresh ginger.
2. Blend until smooth.
3. If desired, add ice cubes and blend again until desired consistency is reached.
4. Pour into glasses and serve immediately.

Nutritional Information (per serving):

- **Carbs:** 25g
- **Sodium:** 20mg
- **Potassium:** 200mg
- **Protein:** 2g

Citrus Berry Burst

Prep Time: 5 minutes | **Cook Time:** 0 minutes | **Servings:** 2

Ingredients:

- 1/2 cup frozen mixed berries (blueberries, strawberries, raspberries)
- 1/2 cup freshly squeezed orange juice
- 1/2 cup unsweetened almond milk
- 1/2 cup plain Greek yogurt
- 1 tablespoon honey
- 1 tablespoon fresh lemon juice
- 1/2 teaspoon grated fresh ginger
- Ice cubes (optional)

Instructions:

1. In a blender, put together the frozen mixed berries, freshly squeezed orange juice, unsweetened almond milk, plain Greek yogurt, honey, fresh lemon juice, and grated fresh ginger.
2. Blend until smooth.
3. If desired, add ice cubes and blend again until desired consistency is reached.
4. Pour into glasses and serve immediately.

Nutritional Information (per serving):

- **Carbs:** 20g
- **Sodium:** 30mg
- **Potassium:** 150mg
- **Protein:** 5g

Mango Berry Tango

Prep Time: 5 minutes | **Cook Time:** 0 minutes | **Servings:** 2

Ingredients:

- 1 cup frozen mango chunks
- 1/2 cup mixed berries (blueberries, strawberries, raspberries)
- 1/2 cup unsweetened coconut water
- 1/2 cup unsweetened almond milk
- 1 tablespoon honey
- 1 tablespoon ground flaxseed
- 1/2 teaspoon grated fresh ginger
- Ice cubes (optional)

Instructions:

1. In a blender, put together the frozen mango chunks, mixed berries, unsweetened coconut water, unsweetened almond milk, honey, ground flaxseed, and grated fresh ginger.
2. Blend until smooth.
3. If desired, add ice cubes and blend again until desired consistency is reached.
4. Pour into glasses and serve immediately.

Nutritional Information (per serving):

- **Carbs:** 25g
- **Sodium:** 25mg
- **Potassium:** 150mg
- **Protein:** 2g

Pineapple Berry Zing

Prep Time: 5 minutes | **Cook Time:** 0 minutes | **Servings:** 2

Ingredients:

- 1 cup frozen pineapple chunks
- 1/2 cup mixed berries (blueberries, strawberries, raspberries)
- 1/2 cup unsweetened coconut water
- 1/2 cup unsweetened almond milk
- 1 tablespoon honey
- 1 tablespoon ground flaxseed
- Ice cubes (optional)

Instructions:

1. In a blender, put together the frozen pineapple chunks, mixed berries, unsweetened coconut water, unsweetened almond milk, honey, and ground flaxseed.
2. Blend until smooth.
3. If desired, add ice cubes and blend again until desired consistency is reached.
4. Pour into glasses and serve immediately.

Nutritional Information (per serving):

- **Carbs:** 25g
- **Sodium:** 20mg
- **Potassium:** 150mg
- **Protein:** 2g

Kiwi Berry Fusion

Prep Time: 5 minutes | **Cook Time:** 0 minutes | **Servings:** 2

Ingredients:

- 2 ripe kiwis, peeled and sliced
- 1/2 cup mixed berries (blueberries, strawberries, raspberries)
- 1/2 cup unsweetened almond milk
- 1/2 cup coconut water
- 1 tablespoon honey
- 1 tablespoon ground flaxseed
- Ice cubes (optional)

Instructions:

1. In a blender, put together the sliced ripe kiwis, mixed berries, unsweetened almond milk, coconut water, honey, and ground flaxseed.
2. Blend until smooth.
3. If desired, add ice cubes and blend again until desired consistency is reached.
4. Pour into glasses and serve immediately.

Nutritional Information (per serving):

- **Carbs:** 20g
- **Sodium:** 20mg
- **Potassium:** 150mg
- **Protein:** 2g

Berry Banana Bliss

Prep Time: 5 minutes | **Cook Time:** 0 minutes | **Servings:** 2

Ingredients:

- 1 cup mixed berries (blueberries, strawberries, raspberries)
- 1 ripe banana, sliced
- 1/2 cup unsweetened almond milk
- 1/2 cup coconut water
- 1 tablespoon honey
- 1 tablespoon ground flaxseed
- Ice cubes (optional)

Instructions:

1. In a blender, put together the mixed berries, sliced ripe banana, unsweetened almond milk, coconut water, honey, and ground flaxseed.
2. Blend until smooth.
3. If desired, add ice cubes and blend again until desired consistency is reached.
4. Pour into glasses and serve immediately.

Nutritional Information (per serving):

- **Carbs:** 25g
- **Sodium:** 20mg
- **Potassium:** 200mg
- **Protein:** 2g

Chapter 4: Green Goodness

Classic Green Revitalizer

Prep Time: 5 minutes | **Cook Time:** 0 minutes | **Servings:** 2

Ingredients:

- 2 cups fresh spinach leaves
- 1 ripe banana, peeled and sliced
- 1 cup chopped pineapple
- 1/2 avocado, peeled and pitted
- 1 tablespoon fresh ginger, peeled and grated
- 1 cup coconut water
- 1 tablespoon chia seeds
- Ice cubes (optional)

Instructions:

1. In a blender, put together the fresh spinach leaves, sliced banana, chopped pineapple, peeled and pitted avocado, grated fresh ginger, and coconut water.
2. Blend until smooth.
3. Add chia seeds and blend for an additional 10-15 seconds.
4. If desired, add ice cubes for a colder consistency and blend again until smooth.
5. Pour the smoothie into glasses and serve immediately.

Nutritional Information (per serving):

- **Carbs:** 32g
- **Sodium:** 60mg
- **Potassium:** 630mg
- **Protein:** 4g

Kale and Kiwi Cleanser

Prep Time: 7 minutes | **Cook Time:** 0 minutes | **Servings:** 2

Ingredients:

- 2 cups kale leaves, stems removed
- 2 kiwis, peeled and diced
- 1 cup unsweetened almond milk
- 1/2 cup frozen blueberries
- 1 tablespoon honey or maple syrup (optional)
- 1 tablespoon flaxseeds

Instructions:

1. Place the kale leaves, diced kiwis, unsweetened almond milk, frozen blueberries, and honey or maple syrup (if using) into a blender.
2. Blend until smooth.
3. Add flaxseeds to the blender and blend for an additional 10-15 seconds.
4. Pour the smoothie into glasses and serve immediately.

Nutritional Information (per serving):

- **Carbs:** 20g
- **Sodium:** 80mg
- **Potassium:** 380mg
- **Protein:** 3g

Spinach Berry Booster

Prep Time: 5 minutes | **Cook Time:** 0 minutes | **Servings:** 2

Ingredients:

- 2 cups fresh spinach leaves

- 1 cup mixed berries (such as strawberries, raspberries, and blueberries)

- 1 ripe banana, peeled and sliced

- 1/2 cup unsweetened almond milk

- 1 tablespoon honey or maple syrup (optional)

- 1 tablespoon ground flaxseeds

Instructions:

1. In a blender, put together the fresh spinach leaves, mixed berries, sliced banana, unsweetened almond milk, and honey or maple syrup (if using).

2. Blend until smooth.

3. Add ground flaxseeds to the blender and blend for an additional 10-15 seconds.

4. Pour the smoothie into glasses and serve immediately.

Nutritional Information (per serving):

- **Carbs:** 25g

- **Sodium:** 70mg

- **Potassium:** 350mg

- **Protein:** 3g

<u>Cucumber Mint Magic</u>

Prep Time: 5 minutes | **Cook Time:** 0 minutes | **Servings:** 2

Ingredients:

- 1 cucumber, peeled and sliced
- 1/2 cup fresh mint leaves
- 1 cup coconut water
- 1 cup frozen pineapple chunks
- 1 tablespoon fresh lime juice
- 1 tablespoon grated fresh ginger
- Ice cubes (optional)

Instructions:

1. In a blender, put together the sliced cucumber, fresh mint leaves, coconut water, frozen pineapple chunks, fresh lime juice, and grated fresh ginger.
2. Blend until smooth.
3. If desired, add ice cubes for a colder consistency and blend again until smooth.
4. Pour the smoothie into glasses and serve immediately.

Nutritional Information (per serving):

- **Carbs:** 20g
- **Sodium:** 80mg
- **Potassium:** 340mg
- **Protein:** 2g

Avocado Green Dream

Prep Time: 5 minutes | **Cook Time:** 0 minutes | **Servings:** 2

Ingredients:

- 1 ripe avocado, peeled and pitted
- 1 cup baby spinach leaves
- 1 cup unsweetened almond milk
- 1 tablespoon honey or maple syrup (optional)
- 1 tablespoon hemp seeds
- 1/2 teaspoon ground cinnamon

Instructions:

1. In a blender, put together the peeled and pitted ripe avocado, baby spinach leaves, unsweetened almond milk, and honey or maple syrup (if using).
2. Blend until smooth.
3. Add hemp seeds and ground cinnamon to the blender and blend for an additional 10-15 seconds.
4. Pour the smoothie into glasses and serve immediately.

Nutritional Information (per serving):

- **Carbs:** 14g
- **Sodium:** 80mg
- **Potassium:** 330mg
- **Protein:** 3g

Green Tea Infusion

Prep Time: 10 minutes | **Cook Time:** 5 minutes | **Servings:** 2

Ingredients:

- 2 cups brewed green tea, cooled
- 1 cup baby spinach leaves
- 1/2 cup frozen mango chunks
- 1/2 cup frozen pineapple chunks
- 1 tablespoon fresh lemon juice
- 1 tablespoon honey or maple syrup (optional)
- Ice cubes (optional)

Instructions:

1. Brew green tea and allow it to cool to room temperature.
2. In a blender, put together the cooled brewed green tea, baby spinach leaves, frozen mango chunks, frozen pineapple chunks, fresh lemon juice, and honey or maple syrup (if using).
3. Blend until smooth.
4. If desired, add ice cubes for a colder consistency and blend again until smooth.
5. Pour the smoothie into glasses and serve immediately.

Nutritional Information (per serving):

- **Carbs:** 20g
- **Sodium:** 10mg
- **Potassium:** 200mg
- **Protein:** 1g

Pineapple Spinach Pleaser

Prep Time: 5 minutes | **Cook Time:** 0 minutes | **Servings:** 2

Ingredients:

- 2 cups fresh spinach leaves

- 1 cup chopped pineapple

- 1/2 cup coconut water

- 1/2 cup unsweetened almond milk

- 1 tablespoon fresh lime juice

- 1 tablespoon grated fresh ginger

- Ice cubes (optional)

Instructions:

1. In a blender, put together the fresh spinach leaves, chopped pineapple, coconut water, unsweetened almond milk, fresh lime juice, and grated fresh ginger.

2. Blend until smooth.

3. If desired, add ice cubes for a colder consistency and blend again until smooth.

4. Pour the smoothie into glasses and serve immediately.

Nutritional Information (per serving):

- **Carbs:** 20g

- **Sodium:** 80mg

- **Potassium:** 290mg

- **Protein:** 2g

<u>Tropical Green Refresher</u>

Prep Time: 5 minutes | **Cook Time:** 0 minutes | **Servings:** 2

Ingredients:

- 2 cups fresh spinach leaves
- 1 cup frozen mango chunks
- 1/2 cup frozen pineapple chunks
- 1/2 cup unsweetened coconut milk
- 1 tablespoon fresh lime juice
- 1 tablespoon shredded coconut (unsweetened)
- Ice cubes (optional)

Instructions:

1. In a blender, put together the fresh spinach leaves, frozen mango chunks, frozen pineapple chunks, unsweetened coconut milk, fresh lime juice, and shredded coconut.
2. Blend until smooth.
3. If desired, add ice cubes for a colder consistency and blend again until smooth.
4. Pour the smoothie into glasses and serve immediately.

Nutritional Information (per serving):

- **Carbs:** 25g
- **Sodium:** 20mg
- **Potassium:** 310mg
- **Protein:** 2g

<u>Matcha Green Energy</u>

Prep Time: 5 minutes | **Cook Time:** 0 minutes | **Servings:** 2

Ingredients:

- 1 teaspoon matcha powder
- 2 cups unsweetened almond milk
- 1 banana, peeled and sliced
- 1 tablespoon honey or maple syrup (optional)
- 1 tablespoon chia seeds
- Ice cubes (optional)

Instructions:

1. In a blender, put together the matcha powder, unsweetened almond milk, sliced banana, and honey or maple syrup (if using).
2. Blend until smooth.
3. Add chia seeds to the blender and blend for an additional 10-15 seconds.
4. If desired, add ice cubes for a colder consistency and blend again until smooth.
5. Pour the smoothie into glasses and serve immediately.

Nutritional Information (per serving):

- **Carbs:** 25g
- **Sodium:** 100mg
- **Potassium:** 250mg
- **Protein:** 3g

Broccoli Blueberry Blend

Prep Time: 5 minutes | **Cook Time:** 0 minutes | **Servings:** 2

Ingredients:

- 1 cup steamed broccoli florets, cooled
- 1 cup frozen blueberries
- 1 banana, peeled and sliced
- 1 cup unsweetened almond milk
- 1 tablespoon honey or maple syrup (optional)
- 1 tablespoon ground flaxseeds

Instructions:

1. Ensure the steamed broccoli florets are cooled before proceeding.
2. In a blender, put together the cooled steamed broccoli florets, frozen blueberries, sliced banana, unsweetened almond milk, and honey or maple syrup (if using).
3. Blend until smooth.
4. Add ground flaxseeds to the blender and blend for an additional 10-15 seconds.
5. Pour the smoothie into glasses and serve immediately.

Nutritional Information (per serving):

- **Carbs:** 25g
- **Sodium:** 80mg
- **Potassium:** 290mg
- **Protein:** 3g

Green Grapes Galore

Prep Time: 5 minutes | **Cook Time:** 0 minutes | **Servings:** 2

Ingredients:

- 2 cups green grapes, washed and stemmed
- 1 cup baby spinach leaves
- 1/2 cup unsweetened coconut water
- 1/2 cup unsweetened almond milk
- 1 tablespoon fresh lime juice
- 1 tablespoon honey or maple syrup (optional)
- Ice cubes (optional)

Instructions:

1. In a blender, put together the washed and stemmed green grapes, baby spinach leaves, unsweetened coconut water, unsweetened almond milk, fresh lime juice, and honey or maple syrup (if using).
2. Blend until smooth.
3. If desired, add ice cubes for a colder consistency and blend again until smooth.
4. Pour the smoothie into glasses and serve immediately.

Nutritional Information (per serving):

- **Carbs:** 20g
- **Sodium:** 40mg
- **Potassium:** 240mg
- **Protein:** 2g

Pear Spinach Paradise

Prep Time: 5 minutes | **Cook Time:** 0 minutes | **Servings:** 2

Ingredients:

- 2 ripe pears, cored and sliced
- 2 cups baby spinach leaves
- 1/2 cup unsweetened almond milk
- 1/2 cup plain Greek yogurt
- 1 tablespoon honey or maple syrup (optional)
- 1 tablespoon ground flaxseeds

Instructions:

1. In a blender, put together the cored and sliced ripe pears, baby spinach leaves, unsweetened almond milk, plain Greek yogurt, and honey or maple syrup (if using).
2. Blend until smooth.
3. Add ground flaxseeds to the blender and blend for an additional 10-15 seconds.
4. Pour the smoothie into glasses and serve immediately.

Nutritional Information (per serving):

- **Carbs:** 30g
- **Sodium:** 60mg
- **Potassium:** 300mg
- **Protein:** 5g

Celery Cilantro Cooler

Prep Time: 5 minutes | **Cook Time:** 0 minutes | **Servings:** 2

Ingredients:

- 2 stalks celery, chopped
- 1/2 cup fresh cilantro leaves
- 1 cup cucumber, peeled and chopped
- 1/2 green apple, cored and chopped
- 1 cup coconut water
- 1 tablespoon fresh lime juice
- Ice cubes (optional)

Instructions:

1. In a blender, put together the chopped celery, fresh cilantro leaves, peeled and chopped cucumber, cored and chopped green apple, coconut water, and fresh lime juice.
2. Blend until smooth.
3. If desired, add ice cubes for a colder consistency and blend again until smooth.
4. Pour the smoothie into glasses and serve immediately.

Nutritional Information (per serving):

- **Carbs:** 15g
- **Sodium:** 150mg
- **Potassium:** 350mg
- **Protein:** 2g

Green Apple Ginger Zest

Prep Time: 5 minutes | **Cook Time:** 0 minutes | **Servings:** 2

Ingredients:

- 2 green apples, cored and chopped
- 1 cup spinach leaves
- 1 tablespoon fresh ginger, peeled and grated
- 1/2 cup unsweetened almond milk
- 1/2 cup coconut water
- 1 tablespoon honey or maple syrup (optional)
- Ice cubes (optional)

Instructions:

1. In a blender, put together the chopped green apples, spinach leaves, grated fresh ginger, unsweetened almond milk, coconut water, and honey or maple syrup (if using).
2. Blend until smooth.
3. If desired, add ice cubes for a colder consistency and blend again until smooth.
4. Pour the smoothie into glasses and serve immediately.

Nutritional Information (per serving):

- **Carbs:** 20g
- **Sodium:** 40mg
- **Potassium:** 280mg
- **Protein:** 2g

<u>Mango Spinach Surprise</u>

Prep Time: 5 minutes | **Cook Time:** 0 minutes | **Servings:** 2

Ingredients:

- 1 ripe mango, peeled and diced
- 2 cups fresh spinach leaves
- 1/2 cup unsweetened coconut water
- 1/2 cup unsweetened almond milk
- 1 tablespoon lime juice
- 1 tablespoon honey or maple syrup (optional)
- Ice cubes (optional)

Instructions:

1. In a blender, put together the diced ripe mango, fresh spinach leaves, unsweetened coconut water, unsweetened almond milk, lime juice, and honey or maple syrup (if using).
2. Blend until smooth.
3. If desired, add ice cubes for a colder consistency and blend again until smooth.
4. Pour the smoothie into glasses and serve immediately.

Nutritional Information (per serving):

- **Carbs:** 25g
- **Sodium:** 40mg
- **Potassium:** 310mg
- **Protein:** 2g

Coconut Kale Craze

Prep Time: 5 minutes | **Cook Time:** 0 minutes | **Servings:** 2

Ingredients:

- 2 cups kale leaves, stems removed
- 1 ripe banana, peeled and sliced
- 1/2 cup coconut milk
- 1/2 cup unsweetened almond milk
- 1 tablespoon coconut oil
- 1 tablespoon honey or maple syrup (optional)
- Ice cubes (optional)

Instructions:

1. In a blender, put together the kale leaves (stems removed), sliced ripe banana, coconut milk, unsweetened almond milk, coconut oil, and honey or maple syrup (if using).
2. Blend until smooth.
3. If desired, add ice cubes for a colder consistency and blend again until smooth.
4. Pour the smoothie into glasses and serve immediately.

Nutritional Information (per serving):

- **Carbs:** 20g
- **Sodium:** 60mg
- **Potassium:** 390mg
- **Protein:** 3g

Pea Protein Power

Prep Time: 5 minutes | **Cook Time:** 0 minutes | **Servings:** 2

Ingredients:

- 2 scoops pea protein powder
- 1 cup unsweetened almond milk
- 1 cup frozen mixed berries
- 1 tablespoon almond butter
- 1 tablespoon honey or maple syrup (optional)
- Ice cubes (optional)

Instructions:

1. In a blender, put together the pea protein powder, unsweetened almond milk, frozen mixed berries, almond butter, and honey or maple syrup (if using).
2. Blend until smooth.
3. If desired, add ice cubes for a colder consistency and blend again until smooth.
4. Pour the smoothie into glasses and serve immediately.

Nutritional Information (per serving):

- **Carbs:** 20g
- **Sodium:** 70mg
- **Potassium:** 200mg
- **Protein:** 15g

Watercress Cucumber Cooler

Prep Time: 5 minutes | **Cook Time:** 0 minutes | **Servings:** 2

Ingredients:

- 2 cups watercress leaves

- 1 cucumber, peeled and chopped

- 1/2 cup coconut water

- 1/2 cup unsweetened almond milk

- 1 tablespoon fresh lemon juice

- 1 tablespoon honey or maple syrup (optional)

- Ice cubes (optional)

Instructions:

1. In a blender, put together the watercress leaves, peeled and chopped cucumber, coconut water, unsweetened almond milk, fresh lemon juice, and honey or maple syrup (if using).

2. Blend until smooth.

3. If desired, add ice cubes for a colder consistency and blend again until smooth.

4. Pour the smoothie into glasses and serve immediately.

Nutritional Information (per serving):

- **Carbs:** 15g

- **Sodium:** 40mg

- **Potassium:** 230mg

- **Protein:** 2g

Chapter 5: Citrus Splash

<u>Orange Turmeric Tonic</u>

Prep Time: 10 minutes | **Cook Time:** 0 minutes | **Servings:** 2

Ingredients:

- 2 large oranges, peeled and segmented
- 1 banana, frozen
- 1 teaspoon turmeric powder
- 1/2 teaspoon ground ginger
- 1/2 teaspoon ground cinnamon
- 1 tablespoon honey (optional)
- 1 cup coconut water
- 1 cup ice cubes

Instructions:

1. In a blender, put together the peeled and segmented oranges, frozen banana, turmeric powder, ground ginger, ground cinnamon, honey (if using), coconut water, and ice cubes.
2. Blend until smooth and creamy.
3. Pour the smoothie into glasses and serve immediately.

Nutritional Information (per serving):

- **Carbs:** 30g
- **Sodium:** 40mg
- **Potassium:** 370mg
- **Protein:** 2g

Lemon Ginger Zinger

Prep Time: 5 minutes | **Cook Time:** 0 minutes | **Servings:** 2

Ingredients:

- 1 cup spinach leaves
- 1 lemon, peeled and seeded
- 1-inch piece of fresh ginger, peeled
- 1/2 cup frozen pineapple chunks
- 1/2 cup frozen mango chunks
- 1 tablespoon chia seeds
- 1 cup unsweetened almond milk
- 1 cup ice cubes

Instructions:

1. In a blender, add the spinach leaves, peeled and seeded lemon, peeled ginger, frozen pineapple chunks, frozen mango chunks, chia seeds, unsweetened almond milk, and ice cubes.

2. Blend until smooth and well combined.

3. Pour the smoothie into glasses and serve immediately.

Nutritional Information (per serving):

- **Carbs:** 20g
- **Sodium:** 70mg
- **Potassium:** 220mg
- **Protein:** 3g

Grapefruit Glow Getter

Prep Time: 5 minutes | **Cook Time:** 0 minutes | **Servings:** 2

Ingredients:

- 1 grapefruit, peeled and segmented
- 1/2 cup frozen strawberries
- 1/2 cup frozen raspberries
- 1/2 cup plain Greek yogurt
- 1 tablespoon flaxseeds
- 1 tablespoon honey (optional)
- 1 cup unsweetened coconut water
- 1 cup ice cubes

Instructions:

1. In a blender, put together the peeled and segmented grapefruit, frozen strawberries, frozen raspberries, plain Greek yogurt, flaxseeds, honey (if using), unsweetened coconut water, and ice cubes.

2. Blend until smooth and creamy.

3. Pour the smoothie into glasses and serve immediately.

Nutritional Information (per serving):

- **Carbs:** 25g
- **Sodium:** 30mg
- **Potassium:** 220mg
- **Protein:** 4g

Lime Basil Blast

Prep Time: 5 minutes | **Cook Time:** 0 minutes | **Servings:** 2

Ingredients:

- 2 limes, peeled and seeded
- 1 cup fresh basil leaves
- 1 cup frozen pineapple chunks
- 1/2 cup frozen mango chunks
- 1 tablespoon hemp seeds
- 1 tablespoon honey (optional)
- 1 cup unsweetened green tea
- 1 cup ice cubes

Instructions:

1. In a blender, add the peeled and seeded limes, fresh basil leaves, frozen pineapple chunks, frozen mango chunks, hemp seeds, honey (if using), unsweetened green tea, and ice cubes.
2. Blend until smooth and well combined.
3. Pour the smoothie into glasses and serve immediately.

Nutritional Information (per serving):

- **Carbs:** 20g
- **Sodium:** 20mg
- **Potassium:** 180mg
- **Protein:** 3g

Citrus Carrot Crush

Prep Time: 5 minutes | **Cook Time:** 0 minutes | **Servings:** 2

Ingredients:

- 2 medium carrots, peeled and chopped
- 1 orange, peeled and segmented
- 1/2 lemon, peeled and seeded
- 1/2 inch piece of fresh ginger, peeled
- 1 cup frozen mango chunks
- 1 tablespoon ground flaxseeds
- 1 tablespoon maple syrup (optional)
- 1 cup unsweetened almond milk
- 1 cup ice cubes

Instructions:

1. In a blender, put together the peeled and chopped carrots, peeled and segmented orange, peeled and seeded lemon, peeled ginger, frozen mango chunks, ground flaxseeds, maple syrup (if using), unsweetened almond milk, and ice cubes.
2. Blend until smooth and creamy.
3. Pour the smoothie into glasses and serve immediately.

Nutritional Information (per serving):

- **Carbs:** 25g
- **Sodium:** 50mg
- **Potassium:** 250mg
- **Protein:** 3g

Pineapple Citrus Sensation

Prep Time: 5 minutes | **Cook Time:** 0 minutes | **Servings:** 2

Ingredients:

- 1 cup fresh pineapple chunks
- 1 orange, peeled and segmented
- 1/2 lemon, peeled and seeded
- 1/2 lime, peeled and seeded
- 1 tablespoon grated fresh turmeric
- 1 tablespoon grated fresh ginger
- 1 tablespoon honey (optional)
- 1 cup unsweetened coconut water
- 1 cup ice cubes

Instructions:

1. In a blender, add the fresh pineapple chunks, peeled and segmented orange, peeled and seeded lemon, peeled and seeded lime, grated fresh turmeric, grated fresh ginger, honey (if using), unsweetened coconut water, and ice cubes.

2. Blend until smooth and well combined.

3. Pour the smoothie into glasses and serve immediately.

Nutritional Information (per serving):

- **Carbs:** 25g
- **Sodium:** 50mg
- **Potassium:** 200mg
- **Protein:** 2g

Mandarin Mango Madness

Prep Time: 5 minutes | **Cook Time:** 0 minutes | **Servings:** 2

Ingredients:

- 2 mandarin oranges, peeled and segmented
- 1 cup frozen mango chunks
- 1/2 cup unsweetened almond milk
- 1 tablespoon ground flaxseeds
- 1 tablespoon grated fresh ginger
- 1 tablespoon honey (optional)
- 1 teaspoon vanilla extract
- 1 cup ice cubes

Instructions:

1. In a blender, put together the peeled and segmented mandarin oranges, frozen mango chunks, unsweetened almond milk, ground flaxseeds, grated fresh ginger, honey (if using), vanilla extract, and ice cubes.
2. Blend until smooth and creamy.
3. Pour the smoothie into glasses and serve immediately.

Nutritional Information (per serving):

- **Carbs:** 25g
- **Sodium:** 40mg
- **Potassium:** 200mg
- **Protein:** 2g

Lemon Lime Loveliness

Prep Time: 5 minutes | **Cook Time:** 0 minutes | **Servings:** 2

Ingredients:

- 1 lemon, peeled and segmented
- 1 lime, peeled and segmented
- 1 cup frozen strawberries
- 1/2 cup frozen blueberries
- 1 tablespoon chia seeds
- 1 tablespoon honey (optional)
- 1 cup unsweetened pomegranate juice
- 1 cup ice cubes

Instructions:

1. In a blender, add the peeled and segmented lemon, peeled and segmented lime, frozen strawberries, frozen blueberries, chia seeds, honey (if using), unsweetened pomegranate juice, and ice cubes.

2. Blend until smooth and well combined.

3. Pour the smoothie into glasses and serve immediately.

Nutritional Information (per serving):

- **Carbs:** 30g
- **Sodium:** 10mg
- **Potassium:** 180mg
- **Protein:** 2g

Citrus Berry Bliss

Prep Time: 5 minutes | **Cook Time:** 0 minutes | **Servings:** 2

Ingredients:

- 1 orange, peeled and segmented
- 1/2 grapefruit, peeled and segmented
- 1 cup mixed berries (such as strawberries, blueberries, raspberries)
- 1 tablespoon ground flaxseeds
- 1 tablespoon honey (optional)
- 1 cup unsweetened cranberry juice
- 1 cup ice cubes

Instructions:

1. In a blender, put together the peeled and segmented orange, peeled and segmented grapefruit, mixed berries, ground flaxseeds, honey (if using), unsweetened cranberry juice, and ice cubes.
2. Blend until smooth and creamy.
3. Pour the smoothie into glasses and serve immediately.

Nutritional Information (per serving):

- **Carbs:** 30g
- **Sodium:** 5mg
- **Potassium:** 160mg
- **Protein:** 2g

Blood Orange Beauty

Prep Time: 5 minutes | **Cook Time:** 0 minutes | **Servings:** 2

Ingredients:

- 2 blood oranges, peeled and segmented
- 1/2 cup frozen raspberries
- 1/2 cup frozen strawberries
- 1 tablespoon ground flaxseeds
- 1 tablespoon honey (optional)
- 1 cup unsweetened pomegranate juice
- 1 cup ice cubes

Instructions:

1. In a blender, add the peeled and segmented blood oranges, frozen raspberries, frozen strawberries, ground flaxseeds, honey (if using), unsweetened pomegranate juice, and ice cubes.
2. Blend until smooth and well combined.
3. Pour the smoothie into glasses and serve immediately.

Nutritional Information (per serving):

- **Carbs:** 30g
- **Sodium:** 5mg
- **Potassium:** 170mg
- **Protein:** 2g

Tangerine Tropical Twist

Prep Time: 5 minutes | **Cook Time:** 0 minutes | **Servings:** 2

Ingredients:

- 2 tangerines, peeled and segmented
- 1/2 cup frozen pineapple chunks
- 1/2 cup frozen mango chunks
- 1 tablespoon hemp seeds
- 1 tablespoon honey (optional)
- 1 cup unsweetened coconut milk
- 1 cup ice cubes

Instructions:

1. In a blender, put together the peeled and segmented tangerines, frozen pineapple chunks, frozen mango chunks, hemp seeds, honey (if using), unsweetened coconut milk, and ice cubes.

2. Blend until smooth and creamy.

3. Pour the smoothie into glasses and serve immediately.

Nutritional Information (per serving):

- **Carbs:** 25g
- **Sodium:** 20mg
- **Potassium:** 180mg
- **Protein:** 2g

Pomelo Passion

Prep Time: 5 minutes | **Cook Time:** 0 minutes | **Servings:** 2

Ingredients:

- 1 pomelo, peeled and segmented
- 1 cup frozen strawberries
- 1/2 cup frozen raspberries
- 1 tablespoon ground flaxseeds
- 1 tablespoon honey (optional)
- 1 cup unsweetened cranberry juice
- 1 cup ice cubes

Instructions:

1. In a blender, add the peeled and segmented pomelo, frozen strawberries, frozen raspberries, ground flaxseeds, honey (if using), unsweetened cranberry juice, and ice cubes.
2. Blend until smooth and well combined.
3. Pour the smoothie into glasses and serve immediately.

Nutritional Information (per serving):

- **Carbs:** 25g
- **Sodium:** 5mg
- **Potassium:** 150mg
- **Protein:** 2g

Lemonade Lavender Lush

Prep Time: 5 minutes | **Cook Time:** 0 minutes | **Servings:** 2

Ingredients:

- 2 lemons, peeled and seeded
- 1 tablespoon dried lavender flowers
- 1 cup frozen blueberries
- 1/2 cup frozen strawberries
- 1 tablespoon chia seeds
- 1 tablespoon honey (optional)
- 1 cup unsweetened almond milk
- 1 cup ice cubes

Instructions:

1. In a blender, add the peeled and seeded lemons, dried lavender flowers, frozen blueberries, frozen strawberries, chia seeds, honey (if using), unsweetened almond milk, and ice cubes.
2. Blend until smooth and creamy.
3. Pour the smoothie into glasses and serve immediately.

Nutritional Information (per serving):

- **Carbs:** 25g
- **Sodium:** 40mg
- **Potassium:** 170mg
- **Protein:** 2g

Citrus Cilantro Cooler

Prep Time: 5 minutes | **Cook Time:** 0 minutes | **Servings:** 2

Ingredients:

- 1 orange, peeled and segmented
- 1 lime, peeled and segmented
- 1/2 cup fresh cilantro leaves
- 1/2 cup frozen pineapple chunks
- 1/2 cup frozen mango chunks
- 1 tablespoon chia seeds
- 1 tablespoon honey (optional)
- 1 cup unsweetened green tea
- 1 cup ice cubes

Instructions:

1. In a blender, put together the peeled and segmented orange, peeled and segmented lime, fresh cilantro leaves, frozen pineapple chunks, frozen mango chunks, chia seeds, honey (if using), unsweetened green tea, and ice cubes.
2. Blend until smooth and well combined.
3. Pour the smoothie into glasses and serve immediately.

Nutritional Information (per serving):

- **Carbs:** 25g
- **Sodium:** 10mg
- **Potassium:** 180mg
- **Protein:** 2g

<u>Citrus Apple Alchemy</u>

Prep Time: 5 minutes | **Cook Time:** 0 minutes | **Servings:** 2

Ingredients:

- 1 orange, peeled and segmented
- 1 apple, cored and chopped
- 1/2 lemon, peeled and seeded
- 1/2 lime, peeled and seeded
- 1 tablespoon grated fresh ginger
- 1 tablespoon honey (optional)
- 1 cup unsweetened apple juice
- 1 cup ice cubes

Instructions:

1. In a blender, add the peeled and segmented orange, chopped apple, peeled and seeded lemon, peeled and seeded lime, grated fresh ginger, honey (if using), unsweetened apple juice, and ice cubes.
2. Blend until smooth and creamy.
3. Pour the smoothie into glasses and serve immediately.

Nutritional Information (per serving):

- **Carbs:** 30g
- **Sodium:** 10mg
- **Potassium:** 190mg
- **Protein:** 1g

Citrus Kale Kicker

Prep Time: 5 minutes | **Cook Time:** 0 minutes | **Servings:** 2

Ingredients:

- 2 oranges, peeled and segmented
- 1 lemon, peeled and seeded
- 1/2 lime, peeled and seeded
- 2 cups fresh kale leaves, stems removed
- 1/2 cup frozen pineapple chunks
- 1/2 cup frozen mango chunks
- 1 tablespoon chia seeds
- 1 tablespoon honey (optional)
- 1 cup unsweetened coconut water
- 1 cup ice cubes

Instructions:

1. In a blender, add the peeled and segmented oranges, peeled and seeded lemon, peeled and seeded lime, fresh kale leaves, frozen pineapple chunks, frozen mango chunks, chia seeds, honey (if using), unsweetened coconut water, and ice cubes.
2. Blend until smooth and well combined.
3. Pour the smoothie into glasses and serve immediately.

Nutritional Information (per serving):

- **Carbs:** 30g
- **Sodium:** 60mg
- **Potassium:** 350mg
- **Protein:** 3g

Orange Bell Pepper Bliss

Prep Time: 5 minutes | **Cook Time:** 0 minutes | **Servings:** 2

Ingredients:

- 2 oranges, peeled and segmented
- 1 yellow bell pepper, seeded and chopped
- 1 cup frozen mango chunks
- 1/2 cup frozen pineapple chunks
- 1 tablespoon grated fresh ginger
- 1 tablespoon honey (optional)
- 1 cup unsweetened coconut water
- 1 cup ice cubes

Instructions:

1. In a blender, add the peeled and segmented oranges, chopped yellow bell pepper, frozen mango chunks, frozen pineapple chunks, grated fresh ginger, honey (if using), unsweetened coconut water, and ice cubes.
2. Blend until smooth and creamy.
3. Pour the smoothie into glasses and serve immediately.

Nutritional Information (per serving):

- **Carbs:** 30g
- **Sodium:** 30mg
- **Potassium:** 270mg
- **Protein:** 2g

Chapter 6: Nutty Nourishment

Almond Joy Delight

Prep Time: 5 minutes | **Cook Time:** 0 minutes | **Servings:** 2

Ingredients:

- 1 ripe banana, sliced and frozen
- 1/4 cup unsweetened shredded coconut
- 1/4 cup raw almonds
- 2 tablespoons cocoa powder
- 1 cup unsweetened almond milk
- 1 tablespoon honey or maple syrup (optional)
- Ice cubes (optional)

Instructions:

1. In a blender, put together the frozen banana slices, shredded coconut, raw almonds, cocoa powder, almond milk, and honey or maple syrup if using.
2. Blend until smooth and creamy.
3. If a thicker consistency is desired, add ice cubes and blend again until smooth.
4. Pour the smoothie into glasses and serve immediately.

Nutritional Information (per serving):

Carbs: 28g | **Sodium:** 80mg | **Potassium:** 430mg | **Protein:** 6g

Anti-inflammatory Smoothie Adaptation:

To adapt the Almond Joy Delight recipe into an anti-inflammatory smoothie with low sodium and potassium content but high antioxidant content, make the following modifications:

Ingredients:

- 1 cup spinach (fresh)
- 1/2 cup blueberries (frozen)
- 1/4 avocado
- 1 tablespoon chia seeds
- 1 teaspoon turmeric
- 1 teaspoon ginger (fresh, grated)
- 1 cup coconut water (unsweetened)

Instructions:

1. In a blender, put together the fresh spinach, frozen blueberries, avocado, chia seeds, turmeric, ginger, and coconut water.
2. Blend until smooth.
3. Pour the smoothie into glasses and serve immediately.

Nutritional Information (per serving):

Carbs: 19g | **Sodium:** 30mg | **Potassium:** 330mg | **Protein:** 3g

Walnut Berry Bonanza

Prep Time: 5 minutes | **Cook Time:** 0 minutes | **Servings:** 2

Ingredients:

- 1 cup mixed berries (such as strawberries, blueberries, raspberries)
- 1/4 cup walnuts
- 1/2 cup Greek yogurt
- 1 tablespoon honey
- 1/2 cup almond milk
- Ice cubes (optional)

Instructions:

1. In a blender, put together the mixed berries, walnuts, Greek yogurt, honey, and almond milk.
2. Blend until smooth.
3. If desired, add ice cubes and blend again until smooth.
4. Pour the smoothie into glasses and serve immediately.

Nutritional Information (per serving):

Carbs: 20g | **Sodium:** 50mg | **Potassium:** 250mg | **Protein:** 7g

Anti-inflammatory Smoothie Adaptation:

To adapt the Walnut Berry Bonanza recipe into an anti-inflammatory smoothie with low sodium and potassium content but high antioxidant content, make the following modifications:

Ingredients:

- 1 cup mixed berries (such as strawberries, blueberries, raspberries) (frozen)
- 1/4 cup walnuts
- 1/2 cup spinach (fresh)
- 1 tablespoon flaxseeds
- 1 teaspoon cinnamon
- 1 cup coconut water (unsweetened)

Instructions:

1. In a blender, put together the frozen mixed berries, walnuts, fresh spinach, flaxseeds, cinnamon, and coconut water.
2. Blend until smooth.
3. Pour the smoothie into glasses and serve immediately.

Nutritional Information (per serving):

Carbs: 15g | **Sodium:** 30mg | **Potassium:** 150mg | **Protein:** 4g

Peanut Butter Banana Bliss

Prep Time: 5 minutes | **Cook Time:** 0 minutes | **Servings:** 2

Ingredients:

- 2 ripe bananas, sliced and frozen
- 2 tablespoons peanut butter
- 1 cup almond milk
- 1 tablespoon honey or maple syrup (optional)
- Ice cubes (optional)

Instructions:

1. In a blender, put together the frozen banana slices, peanut butter, almond milk, and honey or maple syrup if using.
2. Blend until smooth and creamy.
3. If desired, add ice cubes and blend again until smooth.
4. Pour the smoothie into glasses and serve immediately.

Nutritional Information (per serving):

Carbs: 30g | **Sodium:** 80mg | **Potassium:** 450mg | **Protein:** 6g

Anti-inflammatory Smoothie Adaptation:

To adapt the Peanut Butter Banana Bliss recipe into an anti-inflammatory smoothie with low sodium and potassium content but high antioxidant content, make the following modifications:

Ingredients:

- 2 ripe bananas, sliced and frozen
- 2 tablespoons almond butter
- 1 cup kale (fresh)
- 1 tablespoon hemp seeds
- 1 teaspoon turmeric
- 1 teaspoon cinnamon
- 1 cup coconut water (unsweetened)

Instructions:

1. In a blender, put together the frozen banana slices, almond butter, fresh kale, hemp seeds, turmeric, cinnamon, and coconut water.
2. Blend until smooth.
3. Pour the smoothie into glasses and serve immediately.

Nutritional Information (per serving):

Carbs: 20g | **Sodium:** 30mg | **Potassium:** 350mg | **Protein:** 4g

Cashew Cinnamon Swirl

Prep Time: 5 minutes | **Cook Time:** 0 minutes | **Servings:** 2

Ingredients:

- 1/2 cup cashews, soaked in water for at least 2 hours
- 1 ripe banana
- 1 teaspoon cinnamon
- 1 cup unsweetened almond milk
- 1 tablespoon honey or maple syrup (optional)
- Ice cubes (optional)

Instructions:

1. Drain the soaked cashews and add them to a blender.
2. Add the ripe banana, cinnamon, almond milk, and honey or maple syrup if using.
3. Blend until smooth.
4. If desired, add ice cubes and blend again until smooth.
5. Pour the smoothie into glasses and serve immediately.

Nutritional Information (per serving):

Carbs: 25g | **Sodium:** 90mg | **Potassium:** 250mg | **Protein:** 5g

Anti-inflammatory Smoothie Adaptation:

To adapt the Cashew Cinnamon Swirl recipe into an anti-inflammatory smoothie with low sodium and potassium content but high antioxidant content, make the following modifications:

Ingredients:

- 1/2 cup cashews, soaked in water for at least 2 hours
- 1 ripe pear, cored and diced
- 1 teaspoon cinnamon
- 1 cup spinach (fresh)
- 1 tablespoon flaxseeds
- 1 cup coconut water (unsweetened)

Instructions:

1. Drain the soaked cashews and add them to a blender.
2. Add the diced pear, cinnamon, fresh spinach, flaxseeds, and coconut water.
3. Blend until smooth.
4. Pour the smoothie into glasses and serve immediately.

Nutritional Information (per serving):

Carbs: 20g | **Sodium:** 30mg | **Potassium:** 200mg | **Protein:** 4g

Hazelnut Chocolate Indulgence

Prep Time: 5 minutes | **Cook Time:** 0 minutes | **Servings:** 2

Ingredients:

- 1/4 cup hazelnuts
- 2 tablespoons cocoa powder
- 1 ripe banana
- 1 cup unsweetened almond milk
- 1 tablespoon honey or maple syrup (optional)
- Ice cubes (optional)

Instructions:

1. In a blender, put together the hazelnuts, cocoa powder, ripe banana, almond milk, and honey or maple syrup if using.
2. Blend until smooth.
3. If desired, add ice cubes and blend again until smooth.
4. Pour the smoothie into glasses and serve immediately.

Nutritional Information (per serving):

Carbs: 25g | **Sodium:** 90mg | **Potassium:** 300mg | **Protein:** 5g

Anti-inflammatory Smoothie Adaptation:

To adapt the Hazelnut Chocolate Indulgence recipe into an anti-inflammatory smoothie with low sodium and potassium content but high antioxidant content, make the following modifications:

Ingredients:

- 1/4 cup hazelnuts
- 2 tablespoons cocoa powder
- 1/2 cup mixed berries (such as strawberries, blueberries, raspberries) (frozen)
- 1 tablespoon chia seeds
- 1 teaspoon cinnamon
- 1 cup coconut water (unsweetened)

Instructions:

1. In a blender, put together the hazelnuts, cocoa powder, frozen mixed berries, chia seeds, cinnamon, and coconut water.
2. Blend until smooth.
3. Pour the smoothie into glasses and serve immediately.

Nutritional Information (per serving):

Carbs: 20g | **Sodium:** 30mg | **Potassium:** 200mg | **Protein:** 4g

Pistachio Mango Madness

Prep Time: 5 minutes | **Cook Time:** 0 minutes | **Servings:** 2

Ingredients:

- 1/4 cup shelled pistachios
- 1 ripe mango, peeled and diced
- 1 cup unsweetened coconut milk
- 1 tablespoon honey or maple syrup (optional)
- Ice cubes (optional)

Instructions:

1. In a blender, put together the shelled pistachios, diced mango, coconut milk, and honey or maple syrup if using.
2. Blend until smooth.
3. If desired, add ice cubes and blend again until smooth.
4. Pour the smoothie into glasses and serve immediately.

Nutritional Information (per serving):

Carbs: 25g | **Sodium:** 30mg | **Potassium:** 300mg | **Protein:** 4g

Anti-inflammatory Smoothie Adaptation:

To adapt the Pistachio Mango Madness recipe into an anti-inflammatory smoothie with low sodium and potassium content but high antioxidant content, make the following modifications:

Ingredients:

- 1/4 cup shelled pistachios
- 1 ripe mango, peeled and diced
- 1 cup kale (fresh)
- 1 tablespoon flaxseeds
- 1 teaspoon turmeric
- 1 cup coconut water (unsweetened)

Instructions:

1. In a blender, put together the shelled pistachios, diced mango, fresh kale, flaxseeds, turmeric, and coconut water.
2. Blend until smooth.
3. Pour the smoothie into glasses and serve immediately.

Nutritional Information (per serving):

Carbs: 20g | **Sodium:** 30mg | **Potassium:** 200mg | **Protein:** 4g

Macadamia Nut Marvel

Prep Time: 5 minutes | **Cook Time:** 0 minutes | **Servings:** 2

Ingredients:

- 1/4 cup macadamia nuts
- 1 ripe banana
- 1/2 cup pineapple chunks (fresh or frozen)
- 1 cup coconut water (unsweetened)
- 1 tablespoon honey or maple syrup (optional)
- Ice cubes (optional)

Instructions:

1. In a blender, put together the macadamia nuts, ripe banana, pineapple chunks, coconut water, and honey or maple syrup if using.
2. Blend until smooth.
3. If desired, add ice cubes and blend again until smooth.
4. Pour the smoothie into glasses and serve immediately.

Nutritional Information (per serving):

Carbs: 25g | **Sodium:** 30mg | **Potassium:** 300mg |: 3g

Anti-inflammatory Smoothie Adaptation:

To adapt the Macadamia Nut Marvel recipe into an anti-inflammatory smoothie with low sodium and potassium content but high antioxidant content, make the following modifications:

Ingredients:

- 1/4 cup macadamia nuts
- 1 ripe banana
- 1/2 cup blueberries (frozen)
- 1/2 cup spinach (fresh)
- 1 tablespoon chia seeds
- 1 cup green tea (unsweetened)

Instructions:

1. In a blender, put together the macadamia nuts, ripe banana, frozen blueberries, fresh spinach, chia seeds, and green tea.
2. Blend until smooth.
3. Pour the smoothie into glasses and serve immediately.

Nutritional Information (per serving):

Carbs: 20g | **Sodium:** 20mg | **Potassium:** 200mg | **Protein:** 3g

Pecan Pie Pleaser

Prep Time: 5 minutes | **Cook Time:** 0 minutes | **Servings:** 2

Ingredients:

- 1/4 cup pecans
- 1 ripe banana
- 2 tablespoons rolled oats
- 1 tablespoon maple syrup
- 1 cup almond milk
- 1/2 teaspoon vanilla extract
- Ice cubes (optional)

Instructions:

1. In a blender, put together the pecans, ripe banana, rolled oats, maple syrup, almond milk, and vanilla extract.
2. Blend until smooth.
3. If desired, add ice cubes and blend again until smooth.
4. Pour the smoothie into glasses and serve immediately.

Nutritional Information (per serving):

Carbs: 30g | **Sodium:** 90mg | **Potassium:** 270mg | **Protein:** 4g

Anti-inflammatory Smoothie Adaptation:

To adapt the Pecan Pie Pleaser recipe into an anti-inflammatory smoothie with low sodium and potassium content but high antioxidant content, make the following modifications:

Ingredients:

- 1/4 cup pecans
- 1 ripe pear, cored and diced
- 1 tablespoon almond butter
- 1 tablespoon chia seeds
- 1 teaspoon cinnamon
- 1 cup coconut water (unsweetened)

Instructions:

1. In a blender, put together the pecans, diced pear, almond butter, chia seeds, cinnamon, and coconut water.
2. Blend until smooth.
3. Pour the smoothie into glasses and serve immediately.

Nutritional Information (per serving):

Carbs: 20g | **Sodium:** 30mg | **Potassium:** 200mg | **Protein:** 3g

Brazil Nut Berry Blend

Prep Time: 5 minutes | **Cook Time:** 0 minutes | **Servings:** 2

Ingredients:

- 1/4 cup Brazil nuts
- 1 cup mixed berries (such as strawberries, blueberries, raspberries)
- 1 ripe banana
- 1 cup unsweetened almond milk
- 1 tablespoon honey or maple syrup (optional)
- Ice cubes (optional)

Instructions:

1. In a blender, put together the Brazil nuts, mixed berries, ripe banana, almond milk, and honey or maple syrup if using.
2. Blend until smooth.
3. If desired, add ice cubes and blend again until smooth.
4. Pour the smoothie into glasses and serve immediately.

Nutritional Information (per serving):

Carbs: 25g | **Sodium:** 90mg | **Potassium:** 300mg | **Protein:** 4g

Anti-inflammatory Smoothie Adaptation:

To adapt the Brazil Nut Berry Blend recipe into an anti-inflammatory smoothie with low sodium and potassium content but high antioxidant content, make the following modifications:

Ingredients:

- 1/4 cup Brazil nuts
- 1 cup mixed berries (such as strawberries, blueberries, raspberries) (frozen)
- 1/2 cup spinach (fresh)
- 1 tablespoon flaxseeds
- 1 teaspoon turmeric
- 1 cup green tea (unsweetened)

Instructions:

1. In a blender, put together the Brazil nuts, frozen mixed berries, fresh spinach, flaxseeds, turmeric, and green tea.
2. Blend until smooth.
3. Pour the smoothie into glasses and serve immediately.

Nutritional Information (per serving):

Carbs: 20g | **Sodium:** 20mg | **Potassium:** 200mg | **Protein:** 3g

Sunflower Seed Sunshine

Prep Time: 5 minutes | **Cook Time:** 0 minutes | **Servings:** 2

Ingredients:

- 1/4 cup sunflower seeds
- 1 cup pineapple chunks (fresh or frozen)
- 1 ripe banana
- 1 cup coconut water (unsweetened)
- 1 tablespoon honey or maple syrup (optional)
- Ice cubes (optional)

Instructions:

1. In a blender, put together the sunflower seeds, pineapple chunks, ripe banana, coconut water, and honey or maple syrup if using.

2. Blend until smooth.

3. If desired, add ice cubes and blend again until smooth.

4. Pour the smoothie into glasses and serve immediately.

Nutritional Information (per serving):

Carbs: 25g | **Sodium:** 60mg | **Potassium:** 350mg | **Protein:** 4g

Anti-inflammatory Smoothie Adaptation:

To adapt the Sunflower Seed Sunshine recipe into an anti-inflammatory smoothie with low sodium and potassium content but high antioxidant content, make the following modifications:

Ingredients:

- 1/4 cup sunflower seeds
- 1 cup pineapple chunks (fresh or frozen)
- 1/2 cup kale (fresh)
- 1 tablespoon chia seeds
- 1 teaspoon turmeric
- 1 cup green tea (unsweetened)

Instructions:

1. In a blender, put together the sunflower seeds, pineapple chunks, fresh kale, chia seeds, turmeric, and green tea.

2. Blend until smooth.

3. Pour the smoothie into glasses and serve immediately.

Nutritional Information (per serving):

Carbs: 20g | **Sodium:** 20mg | **Potassium:** 200mg | **Protein:** 3g

Sesame Ginger Glow

Prep Time: 5 minutes | **Cook Time:** 0 minutes | **Servings:** 2

Ingredients:

- 1 tablespoon sesame seeds
- 1 inch fresh ginger, peeled and sliced
- 1 ripe banana
- 1 cup unsweetened coconut milk
- 1 tablespoon honey or maple syrup (optional)
- Ice cubes (optional)

Instructions:

1. In a blender, put together the sesame seeds, fresh ginger slices, ripe banana, coconut milk, and honey or maple syrup if using.
2. Blend until smooth.
3. If desired, add ice cubes and blend again until smooth.
4. Pour the smoothie into glasses and serve immediately.

Nutritional Information (per serving):

Carbs: 25g | **Sodium:** 30mg | **Potassium:** 300mg | **Protein:** 3g

Anti-inflammatory Smoothie Adaptation:

To adapt the Sesame Ginger Glow recipe into an anti-inflammatory smoothie with low sodium and potassium content but high antioxidant content, make the following modifications:

Ingredients:

- 1 tablespoon sesame seeds
- 1 inch fresh ginger, peeled and sliced
- 1 cup mixed berries (such as strawberries, blueberries, raspberries) (frozen)
- 1/2 cup spinach (fresh)
- 1 tablespoon flaxseeds
- 1 cup green tea (unsweetened)

Instructions:

1. In a blender, put together the sesame seeds, fresh ginger slices, frozen mixed berries, fresh spinach, flaxseeds, and green tea.
2. Blend until smooth.
3. Pour the smoothie into glasses and serve immediately.

Nutritional Information (per serving):

Carbs: 20g | **Sodium:** 20mg | **Potassium:** 200mg | **Protein:** 3g

Flaxseed Blueberry Boost

Prep Time: 5 minutes | **Cook Time:** 0 minutes | **Servings:** 2

Ingredients:

- 2 tablespoons flaxseeds
- 1 cup blueberries (fresh or frozen)
- 1 ripe banana
- 1 cup unsweetened almond milk
- 1 tablespoon honey or maple syrup (optional)
- Ice cubes (optional)

Instructions:

1. In a blender, put together the flaxseeds, blueberries, ripe banana, almond milk, and honey or maple syrup if using.
2. Blend until smooth.
3. If desired, add ice cubes and blend again until smooth.
4. Pour the smoothie into glasses and serve immediately.

Nutritional Information (per serving):

Carbs: 25g | **Sodium:** 90mg | **Potassium:** 300mg | **Protein:** 3g

Anti-inflammatory Smoothie Adaptation:

To adapt the Flaxseed Blueberry Boost recipe into an anti-inflammatory smoothie with low sodium and potassium content but high antioxidant content, make the following modifications:

Ingredients:

- 2 tablespoons flaxseeds
- 1 cup blueberries (fresh or frozen)
- 1/2 cup kale (fresh)
- 1/2 cup spinach (fresh)
- 1 cup green tea (unsweetened)
- 1 tablespoon honey or maple syrup (optional)

Instructions:

1. In a blender, put together the flaxseeds, blueberries, fresh kale, fresh spinach, and green tea.
2. Blend until smooth.
3. If desired, add honey or maple syrup for sweetness.
4. Pour the smoothie into glasses and serve immediately.

Nutritional Information (per serving):

Carbs: 20g | **Sodium:** 20mg | **Potassium:** 200mg | **Protein:** 3g

Chia Seed Cherry Chill

Prep Time: 5 minutes | **Cook Time:** 0 minutes | **Servings:** 2

Ingredients:

- 2 tablespoons chia seeds
- 1 cup cherries (pitted, fresh or frozen)
- 1 ripe banana
- 1 cup coconut water (unsweetened)
- 1 tablespoon honey or maple syrup (optional)
- Ice cubes (optional)

Instructions:

1. In a blender, put together the chia seeds, cherries, ripe banana, coconut water, and honey or maple syrup if using.
2. Blend until smooth.
3. If desired, add ice cubes and blend again until smooth.
4. Pour the smoothie into glasses and serve immediately.

Nutritional Information (per serving):

Carbs: 25g | **Sodium:** 30mg | **Potassium:** 300mg | **Protein:** 3g

Anti-inflammatory Smoothie Adaptation:

To adapt the Chia Seed Cherry Chill recipe into an anti-inflammatory smoothie with low sodium and potassium content but high antioxidant content, make the following modifications:

Ingredients:

- 2 tablespoons chia seeds
- 1 cup cherries (pitted, fresh or frozen)
- 1/2 cup spinach (fresh)
- 1/2 cup kale (fresh)
- 1 cup green tea (unsweetened)
- 1 tablespoon honey or maple syrup (optional)

Instructions:

1. In a blender, put together the chia seeds, cherries, fresh spinach, fresh kale, and green tea.
2. Blend until smooth.
3. If desired, add honey or maple syrup for sweetness.
4. Pour the smoothie into glasses and serve immediately.

Nutritional Information (per serving):

Carbs: 20g | **Sodium:** 20mg | **Potassium:** 200mg | **Protein:** 3g

Hemp Heart Happiness

Prep Time: 5 minutes | **Cook Time:** 0 minutes | **Servings:** 2

Ingredients:

- 2 tablespoons hemp hearts
- 1 cup mixed berries (such as strawberries, blueberries, raspberries)
- 1 ripe banana
- 1 cup unsweetened almond milk
- 1 tablespoon honey or maple syrup (optional)
- Ice cubes (optional)

Instructions:

1. In a blender, put together the hemp hearts, mixed berries, ripe banana, almond milk, and honey or maple syrup if using.
2. Blend until smooth.
3. If desired, add ice cubes and blend again until smooth.
4. Pour the smoothie into glasses and serve immediately.

Nutritional Information (per serving):

- **Carbs:** 25g
- **Sodium:** 90mg
- **Potassium:** 300mg
- **Protein:** 4g

Anti-inflammatory Smoothie Adaptation:

To adapt the Hemp Heart Happiness recipe into an anti-inflammatory smoothie with low sodium and potassium content but high antioxidant content, make the following modifications:

Ingredients:

- 2 tablespoons hemp hearts
- 1 cup mixed berries (such as strawberries, blueberries, raspberries) (frozen)
- 1/2 cup spinach (fresh)
- 1 tablespoon flaxseeds
- 1 cup green tea (unsweetened)
- 1 tablespoon honey or maple syrup (optional)

Instructions:

1. In a blender, put together the hemp hearts, frozen mixed berries, fresh spinach, flaxseeds, and green tea.
2. Blend until smooth. If desired, add honey or maple syrup for sweetness.
3. Pour the smoothie into glasses and serve immediately.

Nutritional Information (per serving):

Carbs: 20g | **Sodium:** 20mg | **Potassium:** 200mg | **Protein:** 3g

Pumpkin Seed Power

Prep Time: 5 minutes | **Cook Time:** 0 minutes | **Servings:** 2

Ingredients:

- 2 tablespoons pumpkin seeds
- 1 cup diced pumpkin (cooked and cooled)
- 1 ripe banana
- 1 cup unsweetened coconut milk
- 1 tablespoon honey or maple syrup (optional)
- Ice cubes (optional)

Instructions:

1. In a blender, put together the pumpkin seeds, diced pumpkin, ripe banana, coconut milk, and honey or maple syrup if using.
2. Blend until smooth.
3. If desired, add ice cubes and blend again until smooth.
4. Pour the smoothie into glasses and serve immediately.

Nutritional Information (per serving):

- **Carbs:** 25g
- **Sodium:** 30mg
- **Potassium:** 350mg
- **Protein:** 4g

Anti-inflammatory Smoothie Adaptation:

To adapt the Pumpkin Seed Power recipe into an anti-inflammatory smoothie with low sodium and potassium content but high antioxidant content, make the following modifications:

Ingredients:

- 2 tablespoons pumpkin seeds
- 1 cup diced pumpkin (cooked and cooled)
- 1/2 cup kale (fresh)
- 1 tablespoon chia seeds
- 1 teaspoon cinnamon
- 1 cup green tea (unsweetened)

Instructions:

1. In a blender, put together the pumpkin seeds, diced pumpkin, fresh kale, chia seeds, cinnamon, and green tea.
2. Blend until smooth.
3. Pour the smoothie into glasses and serve immediately.

Nutritional Information (per serving):

Carbs: 20g | **Sodium:** 20mg | **Potassium:** 200mg | **Protein:** 3g

Nutty Coconut Craze

Prep Time: 5 minutes | **Cook Time:** 0 minutes | **Servings:** 2

Ingredients:

- 1/4 cup almonds
- 1/4 cup cashews
- 1/4 cup shredded coconut
- 1 ripe banana
- 1 cup unsweetened coconut milk
- 1 tablespoon honey or maple syrup (optional)
- Ice cubes (optional)

Instructions:

1. In a blender, put together the almonds, cashews, shredded coconut, ripe banana, coconut milk, and honey or maple syrup if using.
2. Blend until smooth.
3. If desired, add ice cubes and blend again until smooth.
4. Pour the smoothie into glasses and serve immediately.

Nutritional Information (per serving):

- **Carbs:** 25g
- **Sodium:** 30mg
- **Potassium:** 300mg
- **Protein:** 5g

Anti-inflammatory Smoothie Adaptation:

To adapt the Nutty Coconut Craze recipe into an anti-inflammatory smoothie with low sodium and potassium content but high antioxidant content, make the following modifications:

Ingredients:

- 1/4 cup almonds
- 1/4 cup cashews
- 1/4 cup shredded coconut
- 1/2 cup mixed berries (such as strawberries, blueberries, raspberries) (frozen)
- 1/2 cup kale (fresh)
- 1 cup green tea (unsweetened)

Instructions:

1. In a blender, put together the almonds, cashews, shredded coconut, frozen mixed berries, fresh kale, and green tea.
2. Blend until smooth.
3. Pour the smoothie into glasses and serve immediately.

Nutritional Information (per serving):

Carbs: 20g | **Sodium:** 20mg | **Potassium:** 200mg | **Protein:** 4g

Nutty Apricot Ambrosia

Prep Time: 5 minutes | **Cook Time:** 0 minutes | **Servings:** 2

Ingredients:

- 1/4 cup almonds
- 1/4 cup walnuts
- 1/4 cup dried apricots
- 1 ripe banana
- 1 cup unsweetened almond milk
- 1 tablespoon honey or maple syrup (optional)
- Ice cubes (optional)

Instructions:

1. In a blender, put together the almonds, walnuts, dried apricots, ripe banana, almond milk, and honey or maple syrup if using.
2. Blend until smooth.
3. If desired, add ice cubes and blend again until smooth.
4. Pour the smoothie into glasses and serve immediately.

Nutritional Information (per serving):

Carbs: 25g | **Sodium:** 90mg | **Potassium:** 300mg | **Protein:** 5g

Anti-inflammatory Smoothie Adaptation:

To adapt the Nutty Apricot Ambrosia recipe into an anti-inflammatory smoothie with low sodium and potassium content but high antioxidant content, make the following modifications:

Ingredients:

- 1/4 cup almonds
- 1/4 cup walnuts
- 1/4 cup dried apricots
- 1/2 cup mixed berries (such as strawberries, blueberries, raspberries) (frozen)
- 1/2 cup spinach (fresh)
- 1 cup green tea (unsweetened)

Instructions:

1. In a blender, put together the almonds, walnuts, dried apricots, frozen mixed berries, fresh spinach, and green tea.
2. Blend until smooth.
3. Pour the smoothie into glasses and serve immediately.

Nutritional Information (per serving):

Carbs: 20g | **Sodium:** 20mg | **Potassium:** 200mg | **Protein:** 5g

Nutty Maple Mania

Prep Time: 5 minutes | **Cook Time:** 0 minutes | **Servings:** 2

Ingredients:

- 1/4 cup almonds
- 1/4 cup pecans
- 2 tablespoons maple syrup
- 1 ripe banana
- 1 cup unsweetened almond milk
- Ice cubes (optional)

Instructions:

1. In a blender, put together the almonds, pecans, maple syrup, ripe banana, and almond milk.
2. Blend until smooth.
3. If desired, add ice cubes and blend again until smooth.
4. Pour the smoothie into glasses and serve immediately.

Nutritional Information (per serving):

Carbs: 25g | **Sodium:** 90mg | **Potassium:** 300mg | **Protein:** 4g

Anti-inflammatory Smoothie Adaptation:

To adapt the Nutty Maple Mania recipe into an anti-inflammatory smoothie with low sodium and potassium content but high antioxidant content, make the following modifications:

Ingredients:

- 1/4 cup almonds
- 1/4 cup pecans
- 1 tablespoon flaxseeds
- 1/2 cup mixed berries (such as strawberries, blueberries, raspberries) (frozen)
- 1/2 cup spinach (fresh)
- 1 cup green tea (unsweetened)

Instructions:

1. In a blender, put together the almonds, pecans, flaxseeds, frozen mixed berries, fresh spinach, and green tea.
2. Blend until smooth.
3. Pour the smoothie into glasses and serve immediately.

Nutritional Information (per serving):

Carbs: 20g | **Sodium:** 20mg | **Potassium:** 200mg | **Protein:** 4g

Chapter 7: Spice It Up

Turmeric Ginger Tonic

Prep Time: 5 minutes | **Cook Time:** N/A | **Servings:** 2

Ingredients:

- 1 cup coconut milk (unsweetened)
- 1 ripe banana (frozen)
- 1 tablespoon fresh turmeric (grated)
- 1 tablespoon fresh ginger (grated)
- 1 tablespoon honey
- 1/2 teaspoon ground cinnamon
- 1/2 teaspoon ground black pepper
- 1 tablespoon chia seeds
- 1 tablespoon flaxseed meal
- 1 cup frozen pineapple chunks
- 1/2 cup water

Instructions:

1. In a blender, put in the coconut milk, frozen banana, fresh turmeric, fresh ginger, honey, cinnamon, black pepper, chia seeds, and flaxseed meal.
2. Blend until smooth.
3. Add frozen pineapple chunks and water.
4. Blend again until well combined and smooth.
5. Pour into glasses and serve immediately.

Nutritional Information (per serving):

- **Carbs:** 25g
- **Sodium:** 45mg
- **Potassium:** 300mg
- **Protein:** 3g

Cinnamon Apple Delight

Prep Time: 5 minutes | **Cook Time:** N/A | **Servings:** 2

Ingredients:

- 1 cup almond milk (unsweetened)
- 1 medium apple (cored and diced)
- 1/2 teaspoon ground cinnamon
- 1 tablespoon almond butter
- 1 tablespoon honey
- 1 tablespoon flaxseed meal
- 1/2 teaspoon vanilla extract
- 1 cup ice cubes

Instructions:

1. In a blender, put in the almond milk, diced apple, ground cinnamon, almond butter, honey, flaxseed meal, and vanilla extract.
2. Blend until smooth.
3. Add ice cubes.
4. Blend again until well combined and smooth.
5. Pour into glasses and serve immediately.

Nutritional Information (per serving):

- **Carbs:** 20g
- **Sodium:** 40mg
- **Potassium:** 150mg
- **Protein:** 2g

<u>Ginger Pear Pleaser</u>

Prep Time: 5 minutes | **Cook Time:** N/A | **Servings:** 2

Ingredients:

- 1 cup coconut water
- 2 ripe pears (peeled, cored, and diced)
- 1 tablespoon fresh ginger (grated)
- 1 tablespoon honey
- 1/2 teaspoon ground turmeric
- 1/2 teaspoon ground cinnamon
- 1 tablespoon chia seeds
- 1 tablespoon flaxseed meal
- 1 cup spinach leaves (packed)
- 1 cup ice cubes

Instructions:

1. In a blender, put in the coconut water, diced pears, grated ginger, honey, ground turmeric, ground cinnamon, chia seeds, flaxseed meal, and spinach leaves.
2. Blend until smooth.
3. Add ice cubes.
4. Blend again until well combined and smooth.
5. Pour into glasses and serve immediately.

Nutritional Information (per serving):

- **Carbs:** 22g
- **Sodium:** 35mg
- **Potassium:** 230mg
- **Protein:** 3g

<u>Cardamom Banana Boost</u>

Prep Time: 5 minutes | **Cook Time:** N/A | **Servings:** 2

Ingredients:

- 1 cup almond milk (unsweetened)
- 2 ripe bananas (peeled and sliced)
- 1/2 teaspoon ground cardamom
- 1 tablespoon almond butter
- 1 tablespoon honey
- 1 tablespoon hemp seeds
- 1 tablespoon flaxseed meal
- 1 cup frozen blueberries
- 1 cup ice cubes

Instructions:

1. In a blender, put in the almond milk, sliced bananas, ground cardamom, almond butter, honey, hemp seeds, and flaxseed meal.
2. Blend until smooth.
3. Add frozen blueberries.
4. Blend again until well combined and smooth.
5. Add ice cubes and blend until desired consistency is reached.
6. Pour into glasses and serve immediately.

Nutritional Information (per serving):

- **Carbs:** 30g
- **Sodium:** 50mg
- **Potassium:** 400mg
- **Protein:** 4g

Clove Orange Zest

Prep Time: 5 minutes | **Cook Time:** N/A | **Servings:** 2

Ingredients:

- 1 cup orange juice (freshly squeezed)
- 1 ripe banana (peeled and sliced)
- Zest of 1 orange
- 1/4 teaspoon ground cloves
- 1 tablespoon honey
- 1 tablespoon chia seeds
- 1 tablespoon flaxseed meal
- 1 cup frozen strawberries
- 1 cup ice cubes

Instructions:

1. In a blender, put in the freshly squeezed orange juice, sliced banana, orange zest, ground cloves, honey, chia seeds, and flaxseed meal.
2. Blend until smooth.
3. Add frozen strawberries.
4. Blend again until well combined and smooth.
5. Add ice cubes and blend until desired consistency is reached.
6. Pour into glasses and serve immediately.

Nutritional Information (per serving):

- **Carbs:** 25g
- **Sodium:** 20mg
- **Potassium:** 200mg
- **Protein:** 3g

<u>Cayenne Mango Madness</u>

Prep Time: 5 minutes | **Cook Time:** N/A | **Servings:** 2

Ingredients:

- 1 cup coconut water
- 1 ripe mango (peeled and diced)
- 1/4 teaspoon ground cayenne pepper
- 1 tablespoon honey
- 1 tablespoon hemp seeds
- 1 tablespoon flaxseed meal
- 1 cup kale leaves (packed)
- 1 cup frozen pineapple chunks
- 1 cup ice cubes

Instructions:

1. In a blender, put in the coconut water, diced mango, ground cayenne pepper, honey, hemp seeds, flaxseed meal, and kale leaves.
2. Blend until smooth.
3. Add frozen pineapple chunks.
4. Blend again until well combined and smooth.
5. Add ice cubes and blend until desired consistency is reached.
6. Pour into glasses and serve immediately.

Nutritional Information (per serving):

- **Carbs:** 30g
- **Sodium:** 25mg
- **Potassium:** 300mg
- **Protein:** 3g

Black Pepper Berry Blast

Prep Time: 5 minutes | **Cook Time:** N/A | **Servings:** 2

Ingredients:

- 1 cup almond milk (unsweetened)
- 1 cup mixed berries (such as strawberries, blueberries, and raspberries)
- 1 tablespoon honey
- 1/4 teaspoon ground black pepper
- 1 tablespoon hemp seeds
- 1 tablespoon flaxseed meal
- 1 cup spinach leaves (packed)
- 1 cup frozen mixed berries
- 1 cup ice cubes

Instructions:

1. In a blender, put in the almond milk, mixed berries, honey, ground black pepper, hemp seeds, flaxseed meal, and spinach leaves.
2. Blend until smooth.
3. Add frozen mixed berries.
4. Blend again until well combined and smooth.
5. Add ice cubes and blend until desired consistency is reached.
6. Pour into glasses and serve immediately.

Nutritional Information (per serving):

- **Carbs:** 20g
- **Sodium:** 50mg
- **Potassium:** 200mg
- **Protein:** 3g

Nutmeg Coconut Cream

Prep Time: 5 minutes | **Cook Time:** N/A | **Servings:** 2

Ingredients:

- 1 cup coconut milk (unsweetened)
- 1 ripe banana (peeled and sliced)
- 1/4 teaspoon ground nutmeg
- 1 tablespoon coconut oil
- 1 tablespoon honey
- 1 tablespoon chia seeds
- 1 tablespoon flaxseed meal
- 1 cup frozen mango chunks
- 1 cup ice cubes

Instructions:

1. In a blender, put in the coconut milk, sliced banana, ground nutmeg, coconut oil, honey, chia seeds, and flaxseed meal.
2. Blend until smooth.
3. Add frozen mango chunks.
4. Blend again until well combined and smooth.
5. Add ice cubes and blend until desired consistency is reached.
6. Pour into glasses and serve immediately.

Nutritional Information (per serving):

- **Carbs:** 25g
- **Sodium:** 30mg
- **Potassium:** 250mg
- **Protein:** 3g

Vanilla Spice Sensation

Prep Time: 5 minutes | **Cook Time:** N/A | **Servings:** 2

Ingredients:

- 1 cup almond milk (unsweetened)
- 1 ripe pear (peeled, cored, and diced)
- 1/2 teaspoon ground cinnamon
- 1/4 teaspoon ground nutmeg
- 1 tablespoon honey
- 1 tablespoon almond butter
- 1 tablespoon chia seeds
- 1 tablespoon flaxseed meal
- 1 teaspoon vanilla extract
- 1 cup frozen mixed berries
- 1 cup ice cubes

Instructions:

1. In a blender, put in the almond milk, diced pear, ground cinnamon, ground nutmeg, honey, almond butter, chia seeds, flaxseed meal, and vanilla extract.
2. Blend until smooth.
3. Add frozen mixed berries.
4. Blend again until well combined and smooth.
5. Add ice cubes and blend until desired consistency is reached.
6. Pour into glasses and serve immediately.

Nutritional Information (per serving):

- **Carbs:** 25g
- **Sodium:** 40mg
- **Potassium:** 200mg
- **Protein:** 3g

Rosemary Raspberry Refresher

Prep Time: 5 minutes | **Cook Time:** N/A | **Servings:** 2

Ingredients:

- 1 cup coconut water
- 1 cup fresh raspberries
- 1 tablespoon honey
- 1 tablespoon flaxseed meal
- 1 tablespoon chia seeds
- 1 sprig fresh rosemary
- 1 cup frozen strawberries
- 1 cup ice cubes

Instructions:

1. In a blender, put in the coconut water, fresh raspberries, honey, flaxseed meal, chia seeds, and fresh rosemary sprig.
2. Blend until smooth.
3. Add frozen strawberries.
4. Blend again until well combined and smooth.
5. Add ice cubes and blend until desired consistency is reached.
6. Pour into glasses and serve immediately.

Nutritional Information (per serving):

- **Carbs:** 20g
- **Sodium:** 30mg
- **Potassium:** 150mg
- **Protein:** 2g

Thyme Blueberry Blend

Prep Time: 5 minutes | **Cook Time:** N/A | **Servings:** 2

Ingredients:

- 1 cup almond milk (unsweetened)
- 1 cup fresh blueberries
- 1 tablespoon honey
- 1 tablespoon flaxseed meal
- 1 tablespoon chia seeds
- 2 sprigs fresh thyme
- 1/2 cup frozen spinach
- 1/2 cup frozen blueberries
- 1 cup ice cubes

Instructions:

1. In a blender, put in the almond milk, fresh blueberries, honey, flaxseed meal, chia seeds, and fresh thyme sprigs.
2. Blend until smooth.
3. Add frozen spinach and frozen blueberries.
4. Blend again until well combined and smooth.
5. Add ice cubes and blend until desired consistency is reached.
6. Pour into glasses and serve immediately.

Nutritional Information (per serving):

- **Carbs:** 20g
- **Sodium:** 50mg
- **Potassium:** 200mg
- **Protein:** 3g

Basil Pineapple Pleaser

Prep Time: 5 minutes | **Cook Time:** N/A | **Servings:** 2

Ingredients:

- 1 cup coconut water
- 1 cup fresh pineapple chunks
- 1 tablespoon honey
- 1 tablespoon flaxseed meal
- 1 tablespoon chia seeds
- 3-4 fresh basil leaves
- 1/2 cup frozen mango chunks
- 1/2 cup frozen pineapple chunks
- 1 cup ice cubes

Instructions:

1. In a blender, put in the coconut water, fresh pineapple chunks, honey, flaxseed meal, chia seeds, and fresh basil leaves.
2. Blend until smooth.
3. Add frozen mango chunks and frozen pineapple chunks.
4. Blend again until well combined and smooth.
5. Add ice cubes and blend until desired consistency is reached.
6. Pour into glasses and serve immediately.

Nutritional Information (per serving):

- **Carbs:** 20g
- **Sodium:** 30mg
- **Potassium:** 150mg
- **Protein:** 2g

<u>Minty Melon Magic</u>

Prep Time: 5 minutes | **Cook Time:** N/A | **Servings:** 2

Ingredients:

- 1 cup coconut water

- 1 cup diced honeydew melon

- 1 tablespoon honey

- 1 tablespoon flaxseed meal

- 1 tablespoon chia seeds

- 4-5 fresh mint leaves

- 1/2 cup frozen cucumber slices

- 1/2 cup frozen honeydew melon cubes

- 1 cup ice cubes

Instructions:

1. In a blender, put in the coconut water, diced honeydew melon, honey, flaxseed meal, chia seeds, and fresh mint leaves.

2. Blend until smooth.

3. Add frozen cucumber slices and frozen honeydew melon cubes.

4. Blend again until well combined and smooth.

5. Add ice cubes and blend until desired consistency is reached.

6. Pour into glasses and serve immediately.

Nutritional Information (per serving):

- **Carbs:** 20g

- **Sodium:** 30mg

- **Potassium:** 150mg

- **Protein:** 2g

Coriander Citrus Cleanse

Prep Time: 5 minutes | **Cook Time:** N/A | **Servings:** 2

Ingredients:

- 1 cup orange juice (freshly squeezed)
- 1/2 cup diced pineapple
- 1/2 cup diced mango
- 1 tablespoon honey
- 1 tablespoon flaxseed meal
- 1 tablespoon chia seeds
- 2-3 sprigs fresh coriander (cilantro)
- 1/2 cup frozen mango chunks
- 1/2 cup frozen pineapple chunks
- 1 cup ice cubes

Instructions:

1. In a blender, put in the freshly squeezed orange juice, diced pineapple, diced mango, honey, flaxseed meal, chia seeds, and fresh coriander (cilantro) leaves.
2. Blend until smooth.
3. Add frozen mango chunks and frozen pineapple chunks.
4. Blend again until well combined and smooth.
5. Add ice cubes and blend until desired consistency is reached.
6. Pour into glasses and serve immediately.

Nutritional Information (per serving):

- **Carbs:** 25g
- **Sodium:** 10mg
- **Potassium:** 200mg
- **Protein:** 2g

Fennel Berry Fusion

Prep Time: 5 minutes | **Cook Time:** N/A | **Servings:** 2

Ingredients:

- 1 cup almond milk (unsweetened)
- 1 cup mixed berries (such as strawberries, blueberries, and raspberries)
- 1/2 cup sliced fennel bulb
- 1 tablespoon honey
- 1 tablespoon flaxseed meal
- 1 tablespoon chia seeds
- 1/2 teaspoon ground cinnamon
- 1/2 teaspoon ground ginger
- 1 cup frozen mixed berries
- 1 cup ice cubes

Instructions:

1. In a blender, put in the almond milk, mixed berries, sliced fennel bulb, honey, flaxseed meal, chia seeds, ground cinnamon, and ground ginger.
2. Blend until smooth.
3. Add frozen mixed berries.
4. Blend again until well combined and smooth.
5. Add ice cubes and blend until desired consistency is reached.
6. Pour into glasses and serve immediately.

Nutritional Information (per serving):

- **Carbs:** 20g
- **Sodium:** 50mg
- **Potassium:** 150mg
- **Protein:** 2g

Saffron Strawberry Swirl

Prep Time: 5 minutes | **Cook Time:** N/A | **Servings:** 2

Ingredients:

- 1 cup almond milk (unsweetened)
- 1 cup fresh strawberries
- 1/4 teaspoon saffron threads
- 1 tablespoon honey
- 1 tablespoon flaxseed meal
- 1 tablespoon chia seeds
- 1 teaspoon vanilla extract
- 1 cup frozen strawberries
- 1 cup ice cubes

Instructions:

1. In a blender, put in the almond milk, fresh strawberries, saffron threads, honey, flaxseed meal, chia seeds, and vanilla extract.
2. Blend until smooth.
3. Add frozen strawberries.
4. Blend again until well combined and smooth.
5. Add ice cubes and blend until desired consistency is reached.
6. Pour into glasses and serve immediately.

Nutritional Information (per serving):

- **Carbs:** 20g
- **Sodium:** 50mg
- **Potassium:** 200mg
- **Protein:** 2g

Chili Lime Cooler

Prep Time: 5 minutes | **Cook Time:** N/A | **Servings:** 2

Ingredients:

- 1 cup coconut water
- 1 cup diced cucumber
- 1 tablespoon honey
- Zest and juice of 1 lime
- 1/4 teaspoon chili powder
- 1 tablespoon flaxseed meal
- 1 tablespoon chia seeds
- 1 cup frozen pineapple chunks
- 1 cup ice cubes

Instructions:

1. In a blender, put in the coconut water, diced cucumber, honey, lime zest, lime juice, chili powder, flaxseed meal, and chia seeds.
2. Blend until smooth.
3. Add frozen pineapple chunks.
4. Blend again until well combined and smooth.
5. Add ice cubes and blend until desired consistency is reached.
6. Pour into glasses and serve immediately.

Nutritional Information (per serving):

- **Carbs:** 20g
- **Sodium:** 30mg
- **Potassium:** 200mg
- **Protein:** 2g

Garlic Lime Green

Prep Time: 5 minutes | **Cook Time:** N/A | **Servings:** 2

Ingredients:

- 1 cup coconut water
- 1 cup spinach leaves
- 1/2 avocado, pitted and diced
- 1/2 teaspoon minced garlic
- Juice of 1 lime
- 1 tablespoon honey
- 1 tablespoon flaxseed meal
- 1 tablespoon chia seeds
- 1 cup frozen mango chunks
- 1 cup ice cubes

Instructions:

1. In a blender, put in the coconut water, spinach leaves, diced avocado, minced garlic, lime juice, honey, flaxseed meal, and chia seeds.
2. Blend until smooth.
3. Add frozen mango chunks.
4. Blend again until well combined and smooth.
5. Add ice cubes and blend until desired consistency is reached.
6. Pour into glasses and serve immediately.

Nutritional Information (per serving):

- **Carbs:** 20g
- **Sodium:** 30mg
- **Potassium:** 300mg
- **Protein:** 2g

Chapter 8: Tropical Treats

Pina Colada Paradise

Prep Time: 10 minutes | **Cook Time:** N/A | **Servings:** 2

Ingredients:

- 1 cup frozen pineapple chunks
- 1 ripe banana, sliced
- 1/2 cup coconut milk
- 1/2 cup unsweetened almond milk
- 1 tablespoon honey (optional)
- 1 tablespoon chia seeds
- 1 tablespoon flaxseed meal
- 1/2 teaspoon ground turmeric
- 1/2 teaspoon ground ginger
- 1/4 teaspoon ground cinnamon
- Ice cubes (optional)

Instructions:

1. In a blender, put in the frozen pineapple chunks, sliced banana, coconut milk, almond milk, honey (if using), chia seeds, flaxseed meal, ground turmeric, ground ginger, and ground cinnamon.
2. Blend until smooth and creamy.
3. If desired, add ice cubes to achieve desired consistency and blend again until smooth.
4. Pour into glasses and serve immediately.

Nutritional Information (per serving):

- **Carbs:** 34g
- **Sodium:** 50mg
- **Potassium:** 340mg
- **Protein:** 4g

Tropical Turmeric Twist

Prep Time: 5 minutes | **Cook Time:** N/A | **Servings:** 2

Ingredients:

- 1 cup frozen mango chunks
- 1/2 cup frozen pineapple chunks
- 1 ripe banana, sliced
- 1 cup unsweetened coconut water
- 1 tablespoon fresh lime juice
- 1 teaspoon ground turmeric
- 1 teaspoon grated fresh ginger
- 1 tablespoon honey or maple syrup (optional)
- Ice cubes (optional)

Instructions:

1. In a blender, put in the frozen mango chunks, frozen pineapple chunks, sliced banana, unsweetened coconut water, fresh lime juice, ground turmeric, grated fresh ginger, and honey or maple syrup (if using).
2. Blend until smooth and creamy.
3. If desired, add ice cubes to achieve desired consistency and blend again until smooth.
4. Pour into glasses and serve immediately.

Nutritional Information (per serving):

- **Carbs:** 35g
- **Sodium:** 30mg
- **Potassium:** 340mg
- **Protein:** 2g

Mango Coconut Cream

Prep Time: 5 minutes | **Cook Time:** N/A | **Servings:** 2

Ingredients:

- 1 1/2 cups frozen mango chunks
- 1/2 cup canned light coconut milk
- 1/2 cup unsweetened almond milk
- 1 tablespoon freshly squeezed lime juice
- 1 tablespoon honey or maple syrup (optional)
- 1/2 teaspoon ground turmeric
- 1/2 teaspoon ground cinnamon
- 1 tablespoon shredded unsweetened coconut

Instructions:

1. In a blender, put in the frozen mango chunks, canned light coconut milk, unsweetened almond milk, freshly squeezed lime juice, honey or maple syrup (if using), ground turmeric, and ground cinnamon.
2. Blend until smooth and creamy.
3. Pour into glasses.
4. Sprinkle shredded unsweetened coconut on top before serving.

Nutritional Information (per serving):

- **Carbs:** 30g
- **Sodium:** 20mg
- **Potassium:** 300mg
- **Protein:** 2g

Pineapple Ginger Delight

Prep Time: 5 minutes | **Cook Time:** N/A | **Servings:** 2

Ingredients:

- 2 cups frozen pineapple chunks
- 1 inch piece of fresh ginger, peeled and grated
- 1 cup unsweetened coconut water
- 1 tablespoon honey or maple syrup (optional)
- 1 tablespoon ground flaxseeds
- 1/2 teaspoon ground turmeric
- 1/2 teaspoon ground cinnamon
- Ice cubes (optional)

Instructions:

1. In a blender, put in the frozen pineapple chunks, grated fresh ginger, unsweetened coconut water, honey or maple syrup (if using), ground flaxseeds, ground turmeric, and ground cinnamon.
2. Blend until smooth and creamy.
3. If desired, add ice cubes to achieve desired consistency and blend again until smooth.
4. Pour into glasses and serve immediately.

Nutritional Information (per serving):

- **Carbs:** 30g
- **Sodium:** 20mg
- **Potassium:** 250mg
- **Protein:** 2g

Passionfruit Peach Pleaser

Prep Time: 5 minutes | **Cook Time:** N/A | **Servings:** 2

Ingredients:

- 2 ripe peaches, pitted and sliced
- Pulp of 2 passionfruits
- 1 cup unsweetened almond milk
- 1/2 cup plain Greek yogurt
- 1 tablespoon honey or maple syrup (optional)
- 1 tablespoon ground chia seeds
- 1/2 teaspoon ground turmeric
- 1/2 teaspoon ground ginger
- Ice cubes (optional)

Instructions:

1. In a blender, put in the sliced ripe peaches, pulp of passionfruits, unsweetened almond milk, plain Greek yogurt, honey or maple syrup (if using), ground chia seeds, ground turmeric, and ground ginger.
2. Blend until smooth and creamy.
3. If desired, add ice cubes to achieve desired consistency and blend again until smooth.
4. Pour into glasses and serve immediately.

Nutritional Information (per serving):

- **Carbs:** 24g
- **Sodium:** 40mg
- **Potassium:** 220mg
- **Protein:** 6g

<u>**Guava Berry Blast**</u>

Prep Time: 5 minutes | **Cook Time:** N/A | **Servings:** 2

Ingredients:

- 1 cup guava chunks (fresh or frozen)
- 1/2 cup mixed berries (such as strawberries, blueberries, raspberries)
- 1 ripe banana, sliced
- 1 cup unsweetened cranberry juice
- 1 tablespoon honey or maple syrup (optional)
- 1 tablespoon ground flaxseeds
- 1/2 teaspoon ground turmeric
- 1/2 teaspoon ground cinnamon
- Ice cubes (optional)

Instructions:

1. In a blender, put in the guava chunks, mixed berries, sliced ripe banana, unsweetened cranberry juice, honey or maple syrup (if using), ground flaxseeds, ground turmeric, and ground cinnamon.
2. Blend until smooth and creamy.
3. If desired, add ice cubes to achieve desired consistency and blend again until smooth.
4. Pour into glasses and serve immediately.

Nutritional Information (per serving):

- **Carbs:** 28g
- **Sodium:** 10mg
- **Potassium:** 280mg
- **Protein:** 2g

Kiwi Coconut Bliss

Prep Time: 5 minutes | **Cook Time:** N/A | **Servings:** 2

Ingredients:

- 2 ripe kiwis, peeled and sliced
- 1/2 cup unsweetened coconut milk
- 1/2 cup unsweetened almond milk
- 1 tablespoon honey or maple syrup (optional)
- 1 tablespoon ground chia seeds
- 1/2 teaspoon grated fresh ginger
- 1/2 teaspoon ground turmeric
- 1/4 teaspoon ground cinnamon
- Ice cubes (optional)

Instructions:

1. In a blender, put in the sliced ripe kiwis, unsweetened coconut milk, unsweetened almond milk, honey or maple syrup (if using), ground chia seeds, grated fresh ginger, ground turmeric, and ground cinnamon.
2. Blend until smooth and creamy.
3. If desired, add ice cubes to achieve desired consistency and blend again until smooth.
4. Pour into glasses and serve immediately.

Nutritional Information (per serving):

- **Carbs:** 20g
- **Sodium:** 30mg
- **Potassium:** 240mg
- **Protein:** 2g

Papaya Pineapple Punch

Prep Time: 5 minutes | **Cook Time:** N/A | **Servings:** 2

Ingredients:

- 1 cup diced papaya

- 1 cup diced pineapple

- 1/2 cup unsweetened coconut water

- 1/2 cup unsweetened almond milk

- 1 tablespoon honey or maple syrup (optional)

- 1 tablespoon ground flaxseeds

- 1/2 teaspoon grated fresh ginger

- 1/2 teaspoon ground turmeric

- Ice cubes (optional)

Instructions:

1. In a blender, put in the diced papaya, diced pineapple, unsweetened coconut water, unsweetened almond milk, honey or maple syrup (if using), ground flaxseeds, grated fresh ginger, and ground turmeric.

2. Blend until smooth and creamy.

3. If desired, add ice cubes to achieve desired consistency and blend again until smooth.

4. Pour into glasses and serve immediately.

Nutritional Information (per serving):

- **Carbs:** 26g

- **Sodium:** 20mg

- **Potassium:** 260mg

- **Protein:** 2g

Coconut Lime Cooler

Prep Time: 5 minutes | **Cook Time:** N/A | **Servings:** 2

Ingredients:

- 1 cup coconut water
- Juice of 2 limes
- 1/2 cup unsweetened coconut milk
- 1 tablespoon honey or maple syrup (optional)
- 1 tablespoon shredded unsweetened coconut
- 1/2 teaspoon grated fresh ginger
- Ice cubes (optional)

Instructions:

1. In a blender, put in the coconut water, lime juice, unsweetened coconut milk, honey or maple syrup (if using), shredded unsweetened coconut, and grated fresh ginger.
2. Blend until smooth and creamy.
3. If desired, add ice cubes to achieve desired consistency and blend again until smooth.
4. Pour into glasses and serve immediately.

Nutritional Information (per serving):

- **Carbs:** 16g
- **Sodium:** 20mg
- **Potassium:** 220mg
- **Protein:** 1g

Lychee Berry Bonanza

Prep Time: 5 minutes | **Cook Time:** N/A | **Servings:** 2

Ingredients:

- 1 cup lychee fruits, peeled and pitted
- 1/2 cup mixed berries (such as strawberries, blueberries, raspberries)
- 1 ripe banana, sliced
- 1 cup unsweetened almond milk
- 1 tablespoon honey or maple syrup (optional)
- 1 tablespoon ground flaxseeds
- 1/2 teaspoon ground turmeric
- 1/2 teaspoon ground ginger
- Ice cubes (optional)

Instructions:

1. In a blender, put in the peeled and pitted lychee fruits, mixed berries, sliced ripe banana, unsweetened almond milk, honey or maple syrup (if using), ground flaxseeds, ground turmeric, and ground ginger.
2. Blend until smooth and creamy.
3. If desired, add ice cubes to achieve desired consistency and blend again until smooth.
4. Pour into glasses and serve immediately.

Nutritional Information (per serving):

- **Carbs:** 28g
- **Sodium:** 20mg
- **Potassium:** 250mg
- **Protein:** 2g

Dragon Fruit Dream

Prep Time: 5 minutes | **Cook Time:** N/A | **Servings:** 2

Ingredients:

- 1 dragon fruit, peeled and diced
- 1 cup frozen strawberries
- 1/2 cup unsweetened coconut water
- 1/2 cup unsweetened almond milk
- 1 tablespoon honey or maple syrup (optional)
- 1 tablespoon ground chia seeds
- 1/2 teaspoon ground turmeric
- 1/2 teaspoon ground ginger
- Ice cubes (optional)

Instructions:

1. In a blender, put in the diced dragon fruit, frozen strawberries, unsweetened coconut water, unsweetened almond milk, honey or maple syrup (if using), ground chia seeds, ground turmeric, and ground ginger.
2. Blend until smooth and creamy.
3. If desired, add ice cubes to achieve desired consistency and blend again until smooth.
4. Pour into glasses and serve immediately.

Nutritional Information (per serving):

- **Carbs:** 25g
- **Sodium:** 20mg
- **Potassium:** 260mg
- **Protein:** 2g

Starfruit Sensation

Prep Time: 5 minutes | **Cook Time:** N/A | **Servings:** 2

Ingredients:

- 1 ripe starfruit, sliced

- 1 cup frozen mango chunks

- 1/2 cup unsweetened coconut water

- 1/2 cup unsweetened almond milk

- 1 tablespoon honey or maple syrup (optional)

- 1 tablespoon ground flaxseeds

- 1/2 teaspoon ground turmeric

- 1/2 teaspoon ground cinnamon

- Ice cubes (optional)

Instructions:

1. In a blender, put in the sliced ripe starfruit, frozen mango chunks, unsweetened coconut water, unsweetened almond milk, honey or maple syrup (if using), ground flaxseeds, ground turmeric, and ground cinnamon.

2. Blend until smooth and creamy.

3. If desired, add ice cubes to achieve desired consistency and blend again until smooth.

4. Pour into glasses and serve immediately.

Nutritional Information (per serving):

- **Carbs:** 26g

- **Sodium:** 20mg

- **Potassium:** 260mg

- **Protein:** 2g

Jackfruit Java Jolt

Prep Time: 5 minutes | **Cook Time:** N/A | **Servings:** 2

Ingredients:

- 1 cup diced jackfruit
- 1 ripe banana, sliced
- 1 cup chilled brewed coffee
- 1/2 cup unsweetened almond milk
- 1 tablespoon honey or maple syrup (optional)
- 1 tablespoon cocoa powder
- 1/2 teaspoon ground cinnamon
- Ice cubes (optional)

Instructions:

1. In a blender, put in the diced jackfruit, sliced ripe banana, chilled brewed coffee, unsweetened almond milk, honey or maple syrup (if using), cocoa powder, and ground cinnamon.
2. Blend until smooth and creamy.
3. If desired, add ice cubes to achieve desired consistency and blend again until smooth.
4. Pour into glasses and serve immediately.

Nutritional Information (per serving):

- **Carbs:** 25g
- **Sodium:** 20mg
- **Potassium:** 220mg
- **Protein:** 2g

Coconut Banana Breeze

Prep Time: 5 minutes | **Cook Time:** N/A | **Ingredients:**

- 2 ripe bananas, sliced
- 1/2 cup unsweetened coconut milk
- 1/2 cup unsweetened almond milk
- 1 tablespoon honey or maple syrup (optional)
- 1 tablespoon shredded unsweetened coconut
- 1/2 teaspoon ground turmeric
- 1/2 teaspoon ground cinnamon
- Ice cubes (optional)

Instructions:

1. In a blender, put in the sliced ripe bananas, unsweetened coconut milk, unsweetened almond milk, honey or maple syrup (if using), shredded unsweetened coconut, ground turmeric, and ground cinnamon.
2. Blend until smooth and creamy.
3. If desired, add ice cubes to achieve desired consistency and blend again until smooth.
4. Pour into glasses and serve immediately.

Nutritional Information (per serving):

- **Carbs:** 24g
- **Sodium:** 20mg
- **Potassium:** 250mg
- **Protein:** 2g

Mango Papaya Passion

Prep Time: 5 minutes | **Cook Time:** N/A | **Servings:** 2

Ingredients:

- 1 cup diced mango
- 1 cup diced papaya
- 1/2 cup unsweetened almond milk
- 1/2 cup coconut water
- 1 tablespoon honey or maple syrup (optional)
- 1 tablespoon ground flaxseeds
- 1/2 teaspoon grated fresh ginger
- 1/2 teaspoon ground turmeric
- Ice cubes (optional)

Instructions:

1. In a blender, put in the diced mango, diced papaya, unsweetened almond milk, coconut water, honey or maple syrup (if using), ground flaxseeds, grated fresh ginger, and ground turmeric.
2. Blend until smooth and creamy.
3. If desired, add ice cubes to achieve desired consistency and blend again until smooth.
4. Pour into glasses and serve immediately.

Nutritional Information (per serving):

- **Carbs:** 25g
- **Sodium:** 15mg
- **Potassium:** 250mg
- **Protein:** 2g

Kiwi Pineapple Perfection

Prep Time: 5 minutes | **Cook Time:** N/A | **Servings:** 2

Ingredients:

- 2 kiwis, peeled and sliced
- 1 cup diced pineapple
- 1/2 cup unsweetened coconut water
- 1/2 cup unsweetened almond milk
- 1 tablespoon honey or maple syrup (optional)
- 1 tablespoon ground chia seeds
- 1/2 teaspoon ground turmeric
- 1/2 teaspoon ground ginger
- Ice cubes (optional)

Instructions:

1. In a blender, put in the sliced kiwis, diced pineapple, unsweetened coconut water, unsweetened almond milk, honey or maple syrup (if using), ground chia seeds, ground turmeric, and ground ginger.
2. Blend until smooth and creamy.
3. If desired, add ice cubes to achieve desired consistency and blend again until smooth.
4. Pour into glasses and serve immediately.

Nutritional Information (per serving):

- **Carbs:** 25g
- **Sodium:** 20mg
- **Potassium:** 250mg
- **Protein:** 2g

Passionfruit Orange Oasis

Prep Time: 5 minutes | **Cook Time:** N/A | **Servings:** 2

Ingredients:

- 2 passionfruits, pulp removed
- Juice of 2 oranges
- 1/2 cup unsweetened almond milk
- 1/2 cup coconut water
- 1 tablespoon honey or maple syrup (optional)
- 1 tablespoon ground flaxseeds
- 1/2 teaspoon ground turmeric
- 1/2 teaspoon ground ginger
- Ice cubes (optional)

Instructions:

1. In a blender, put in the passionfruit pulp, juice of oranges, unsweetened almond milk, coconut water, honey or maple syrup (if using), ground flaxseeds, ground turmeric, and ground ginger.

2. Blend until smooth and creamy.

3. If desired, add ice cubes to achieve desired consistency and blend again until smooth.

4. Pour into glasses and serve immediately.

Nutritional Information (per serving):

- **Carbs:** 20g
- **Sodium:** 25mg
- **Potassium:** 200mg
- **Protein:** 2g

Tropical Basil Bliss

Prep Time: 5 minutes | **Cook Time:** N/A | **Servings:** 2

Ingredients:

- 1 cup diced pineapple
- 1 cup diced mango
- 1/2 cup unsweetened coconut water
- 1/2 cup unsweetened almond milk
- 1 tablespoon honey or maple syrup (optional)
- 1 tablespoon fresh basil leaves
- 1 tablespoon ground flaxseeds
- 1/2 teaspoon ground turmeric
- 1/2 teaspoon ground ginger
- Ice cubes (optional)

Instructions:

1. In a blender, put in the diced pineapple, diced mango, unsweetened coconut water, unsweetened almond milk, honey or maple syrup (if using), fresh basil leaves, ground flaxseeds, ground turmeric, and ground ginger.
2. Blend until smooth and creamy.
3. If desired, add ice cubes to achieve desired consistency and blend again until smooth.
4. Pour into glasses and serve immediately.

Nutritional Information (per serving):

- **Carbs:** 25g
- **Sodium:** 20mg
- **Potassium:** 250mg
- **Protein:** 2g

Chapter 9: Key Tips for Sustaining Anti-Inflammatory Juicing Long-Term

Adopting anti-inflammatory juicing as a long-term practice can profoundly affect your health and wellness. However, maintaining this habit requires consistency, creativity, and strategic thinking. Here are some essential tips to help you gradually adopt anti-inflammatory juicing into your lifestyle:

1. Establish a Routine

Establishing a consistent routine is essential for incorporating juicing into your daily life. Establish regular intervals throughout your day or week solely devoted to juicing. Having a set schedule can help establish it as a long-term habit, whether it's a morning juicing routine to start your day or an evening ritual to relax and unwind.

2. Plan and Prep Ahead

Being well-prepared is crucial for maintaining any healthy habit. Plan your juices and smoothies for the week ahead and prepare your ingredients in advance. Ensure that your fruits and vegetables are properly prepared and stored in the refrigerator or freezer for convenient use whenever necessary. Preparing ahead of time helps avoid the urge to skip juicing when pressed for time.

3. Simplicity is Crucial

Although it can be exciting to try out new recipes, opting for simplicity is often a more sustainable approach. Begin with simple, straightforward juices and smoothies made with just a few ingredients. As you get more accustomed to the process, you can gradually incorporate more complex recipes.

4. Variety is Key

It's important to regularly switch up your ingredients to prevent monotony and maximize nutritional variety. Experiment with various fresh ingredients, including seasonal produce, to create unique flavor combinations. Different types of food keep things exciting and offer a broader range of anti-inflammatory compounds.

5. Listen to Your Body

Be mindful of how your body reacts to various juices and smoothies. Every individual has their distinct nutritional requirements and sensitivities. If a specific ingredient doesn't agree with you, adjust your recipes as needed. Being in tune with your body is vital to making your juicing routine enjoyable and beneficial.

6. Stay Informed and Motivated

Stay informed about the benefits of incorporating anti-inflammatory foods into your diet and explore the latest juicing techniques. Stay informed and motivated by following reputable health blogs, joining juicing communities, and reading books on the subject. Having accurate knowledge empowers you to make well-informed choices and stay dedicated to your juicing journey.

7. Balance with Whole Foods

Although juicing is an excellent method for obtaining concentrated nutrients, it's crucial to complement it with whole foods for a well-rounded diet. Your diet must have a diverse range of whole fruits, vegetables, grains, proteins, and healthy fats. This balance offers a complete range of nutrients to combat inflammation and promote overall well-being.

8. Invest in Quality Equipment

A reliable, superb blender or juicer can significantly enhance the convenience and pleasure of juicing. Invest in equipment that suits your needs and budget. High-quality tools not only improve the texture and flavor of your juices but also make the process more efficient and enjoyable.

By incorporating these essential tips into your routine, you can maintain a long-term commitment to anti-inflammatory juicing. Consistency, planning, variety, and knowledge are vital to keeping any healthy habit. Incorporating these activities into your daily routine can provide you with the long-term benefits of anti-inflammatory juicing.

Conclusion

Beginning an anti-inflammatory juicing journey is a decisive step toward improving your overall health. By incorporating nutrient-rich, inflammation-fighting ingredients into your daily routine, you can enjoy a wide range of benefits, including a lower risk of chronic diseases, improved immune function, and better digestive health.

This cookbook delves into the basics of inflammation, highlights the benefits of an anti-inflammatory diet, and offers a range of delectable smoothie recipes designed to help you achieve your health objectives. We have also provided valuable advice on choosing the perfect ingredients, creating a harmonious blend of flavors and nutrients, and maintaining the ideal storage and preparation methods for your smoothies.

It's essential to maintain this healthy habit over time by being consistent and trying out new smoothie recipes every once in a while, to keep things exciting. Establish a routine, plan ahead, keep your recipes simple yet varied, and always listen to your body's needs. By incorporating these nutritious drinks into your routine, you can experience their immediate benefits and develop a lifestyle that promotes long-term wellness.

Thank you for joining us on this journey toward better health. May your acquired knowledge and the recipes in this book inspire you to make anti-inflammatory juicing an exciting and essential part of your daily routine. Cheers to a healthier and happier you!

Recipes Index

S

T

V

W